W9-CKQ-001

IS THERE A DUTY TO DIE?

Reflective Bioethics Series

IS THERE A DUTY TO DIE?

and Other Essays in Bioethics

John Hardwig

with **Nat Hentoff**

Daniel Callahan

Felicia Cohn and Joanne Lynn

Larry R. Churchill

Routledge

New York and London

Published in 2000 by
Routledge
29 West 35th Street
New York, NY 10001

Published in Great Britain by
Routledge
11 New Fetter Lane
London EC4P 4EE

10 9 8 7 6 5 4 3 2 1

Library of Congress Cataloging-in-Publication Data

Hardwig, John.
   Is There a Duty to Die? : and other essays in bioethics / by John Hardwig,
with Nat Hentoff . . . [et al.].
      p.   cm.
   Includes bibliographical references and index.
   ISBN 0-415-92241-0 (hb).—ISBN 0-415-92242-9 (pb)
   1. Death—Moral and ethical aspects. 2. Medical Ethics.
I. Hentoff, Nat. II. Title.
R725.5.H37 1999
174'.24—dc21
                                                        99-13222
                                                        CIP

For Mary

Contents

Acknowledgments

1. "In Search of an Ethics of Personal Relationships" in Graham, G. & Lafollette, H., *Person to Person* (Temple University Press, 1988), 63–81.

2. "What About the Family?—The Role of Family Interests in Medical Decision Making," *Hastings Center Reports*, 20 [March/April] (1990), 5–10.

3. "The Problem of Proxies with Interests of Their Own: Toward a Better Theory of Proxy Decisions," *Journal of Clinical Ethics*, 4, (1993), 20–7.

4. "SUPPORT and the Invisible Family," Special Supplement, *Hastings Center Report*, 25, no. 6, (1995), S23–S25.

5. "Elder Abuse, Ethics, and Context" in Cebik, L.B., Edwards, R.B. et al., eds., *Violence, Neglect, and the Elderly* (JAI Press, 1996), 41–55.

6. "Dying at the Right Time: Reflections on (Un)assisted Suicide" in LaFollette, H., ed., *Ethics in Practice* (Blackwell, 1996), 53–65.

7. "Autobiography, Biography, and Narrative Ethics" in Nelson, H., ed., *Stories and Their Limits: Narrative Approaches to Bioethics* (Routledge, 1997), 50–64.

8. "Is There a Duty to Die?" *Hastings Center Report*, 27, no. 2, (1997), 34–42.

9. Nat Hentoff, "Duty to Die?" *The Washington Post*, May 31, 1997.

Introduction

I found myself watching the families. I was a college teacher trained as a philosopher, and now I was charged with the task of trying to turn myself into a bioethicist. I was unfamiliar with hospitals and uncomfortable in them. The medical jargon baffled me. I had no clinical eye to tell how the patient was doing. The new and largely undefined role added to my discomfort. I knew that I was supposed to help doctors with the ethical aspects of their decisions, but I couldn't even understand their conversations about those decisions.

The attention of the physicians and medical students I accompanied on teaching rounds was focused on the patient, and especially on the patient's illness. They talked mainly about the clinical variables that might provide the keys to restoring health, or at least combating the effects of incurable illness. The activities of other health care professionals—nurses, therapists, technicians—also centered on the patient.

Most of the time, doctors and hospital staff do not pay much attention to the patients' families. Yet even to my untrained eye, it was evident that a serious illness or death represents a profound crisis for everyone in the family. Death and dying are often much more difficult for the survivors than for the dying patient. Family members also sometimes suffer more than the patient from the patient's debilitating or chronic illness. Families are torn apart by disagreements over treatment options, and I could easily imagine those rifts echoing through the family for decades—"I'm still not speaking to Joe after what he did to Mom." I saw families struggling to cope with the consequences of decisions doctors and patients made—decisions that would often seriously compromise the lives of the patient's loved ones, sometimes even without substantial benefit to the patient.

This focus on the patient usually means that the discharge of a patient is thought of as the end of the story—she is gone, no longer a patient here, no longer in our care. A discharged patient is a success, a happy ending to the story. But a discharge is seldom the end of the story. Especially not now, when patients are frequently discharged still battling chronic illnesses rather than cured. Although a loved one in the hospital might once have been a brief disruption of family life, today the ramifications of decisions made in the hospital more frequently continue to unfold long afterward in the life of a family, sometimes for decades. Even when the patient dies, that is still not the end of the story. The death of a loved one and the *way* she died may rearrange the life of a family for a year or more. Indeed, a death in the family can haunt family members for the rest of their lives.

Hospitals—and most hospital physicians—are not very good at dealing with family crises or responding to the needs of those who love and care for the patient. Family members are "visitors," not patients, so the staff often does not feel responsible for caring for them. The brief conversations physicians have with "the family" are generally social courtesies that serve only to inform family members about how the patient is doing medically. Sometimes these brief encounters are too compressed and not honest enough to ever be informative. Families are normally silenced—they are not consulted except when the patient is incapable of speaking for herself. Even then, family members are asked only what the patient would have wanted—never what they themselves want. What this illness or the treatment of it will mean for their lives is considered irrelevant.

I asked the hospital chaplain one day whether he knew of families that had been seriously damaged by what had been done in the hospital. "Sure," he replied, "lots of them." Then I asked whether he knew of families that had been made whole, stronger, or healthier by what was done in the hospital. He thought for awhile, "I can't think of any," he said. "None come to mind." This, too, may be a result of the focus on the patient and on the disease of the patient.

When I left the hospital, I would return to my office to try to get myself up to speed in the literature of bioethics. I was surprised to find that families were also ignored and silenced by those writing in bioethics. The routine dismissal of the interests of the family I had witnessed in the hospital is sanctioned and promoted in the literature of bioethics.

Bioethicists almost unanimously advocate a "patient-centered

2

ethics," an ethics that claims that only *the patient's* interests and values are to be considered in medical treatment decisions. That makes sense when only the patient is (significantly) affected by a medical treatment decision. But that's often not the case. Why, then, are the rest of the family's interests not to enter at all into the moral equation, and certainly not if they conflict with what's best for the patient? How can it be ethical to consider only what's best for one—the patient—when decisions are made that will dramatically alter the lives of all members of a family?

I wondered whether anyone else was watching the families and thinking about what doctors and hospitals are doing to them.[1] I knew that sometimes the practice of medicine is ethically better than our theories of medical ethics. Some physicians, especially primary care physicians in rural areas, pay close attention to the impact of treatment options on their patients' families. Here is one doctor's account of how health care decisions were made 50 years ago in rural Nebraska:

> The entire family used to gather around grandmother's bed and discuss whether to send grandma to the hospital or Junior to college. If she was able, grandma herself would sometimes participate in this discussion. I can see nothing demeaning or degrading to grandma in such discussions.

When I heard this story, I was struck by the moral sensitivity and wisdom displayed—here, in practice, was an ethic attuned to the inseparability of the lives of the members of families and to the implications of treatment decisions for the patient's loved ones. But it was hard to imagine such conversations in a modern hospital, or physicians participating willingly in them. And I could find nothing in either the traditional ethics of medicine or contemporary bioethics that would explain or justify such discussions and decisions.

A patient-centered ethics is, I sensed, fundamentally at odds with the ethics of families.[2] In a family, the working assumption is that any major decision will inevitably affect the lives of all members of the family. So the interests and well-being of all members of the family must be considered and weighed in making *any* major decision. In a family, no one's interests are irrelevant, and no one's interests are to trump the rest. No one—except for a very short period of time—should be the exclusive focus of the efforts of an entire family. Because lives within a family are deeply intertwined, there will inevitably be complex trade-offs and careful attempts to juggle or harmonize the different interests of everyone. Attempts at compromise, as well as sacrifices, are needed all around. Loyalty to the rest is required of all. Finally, everyone in the family must be allowed to speak, not only of what she herself has at stake in a decision, but also about her vision of what would be best for the entire family. What each has to say must be heard; it must help shape any final decision.

What happened? How could the impact of medical treatment on the patient's loved ones and families have been overlooked and ignored or dismissed as morally irrelevant? How could families be so routinely silenced?

What I suspect happened is this. When philosophers and theologians became bioethicists and started going into hospitals, they succumbed to the focus on the patient and the health-related concerns of the hospital. They saw themselves as developing an ethics for doctors and began this task with an ethical analysis of the doctor-patient relationship. Focusing on this relationship, it was easy to fall into the unspoken assumption that the doctor and patient are the only two people in the picture, hence the only people who belong in the moral equation. In fact, the families often were not part of the picture—they were usually not present when decisions were made, and patient confidentiality could be invoked to make sure they would not be present. They were clearly peripheral to the focus of the hospital; they could be ignored, they *were* ignored. Bioethicists could also fall quite naturally into thinking of discharge as the end of "the case," and if discharge is the end of the matter, families may appear not to have all that much at stake in treatment decisions.

So bioethicists fell into thinking in terms of the ethics of a dyad, the doctor and the patient. The ethics of this dyad seemed straightforward: The doctor is to serve the interests of the patient. The central issue then became: Who defines the interests of the patient? Bioethicists saw rampant paternalism in the doctor-patient relationship, with doctors making far too many decisions for patients. So they sought to empower patients by helping them recover the right to define their own interests, goals, and values and make treatment decisions on the basis of their own perceptions of what is best for them. "Let the patient decide" became the slogan of bioethics, patient autonomy its watchword. "Whose life is it, anyway?" bioethicists asked rhetorically, as if the lives of family members were separable and treatment decisions would affect no one but the patient.

This patient-centered bioethics fell neatly into line with the official ethics of traditional medicine. The Hippocratic oath states, "Whatever house I enter, I will enter for the benefit of the sick." Moreover, doctors, nurses, and other health professionals are all trained to think of themselves as advocates for their patients. So bioethicists could say to health professionals, "Retain your patient-centered ethics and your patient advocacy. You are right to serve the interests of your patient exclusively. Only recognize that the patient is normally more knowledgeable about her own interests than we are."

That is a simple, manageable message. A patient-centered ethics also greatly simplified the task of bioethicists. All the new moral problems of medicine are much easier if only the patient's interests are considered relevant.

In the last 10 years or so, the powerful "cost-containment" movement in medicine has forced the expansion of the doctor-patient dyad into a triad that now includes the interests of "third-party payers." Since someone must pay for all this health care, bioethicists and physicians have reluctantly admitted that the interests of the payers—employers, insurance companies, the government, HMOs—are morally relevant. Just how considerations of cost to third-party payers are to be considered in the ethics of health care is currently *the* question of bioethics.

But through all this, the family is still left out of consideration. Strangely, only monetary costs—not human costs—are considered morally relevant to medical treatment decisions, and then only the monetary costs to an employer, the government, an insurer, an HMO, the hospital, or the physician. When the family must pay, the costs—both financial and human—again vanish from the moral equation. Worse yet, costs are increasingly being shifted onto families, as patients are discharged from hospitals "quicker and sicker." This practice substitutes care by family members for professional care, and the financial costs, too, are often shifted onto families. Most families have little ability to pay these costs, and they often "pay" in real sacrifices in the quality of their lives—unrelieved caregiving, social isolation, depleted savings, and lost careers.

If we do not think about families, we may not even fully acknowledge the sacrifices our cost-containment effort imposes on them. We see only that it saves money for employers, insurers, and hospitals; our only concern is that *patients* may not do quite as well with home care.

Seventeen years later, I am still watching the families. The deep conviction that we must not lose sight of patients' families dovetailed with my interest in thinking about the ethics of personal relationships—love, friendships, relationships, and families—and the essays that make up this volume were born. They record my attempt to work toward a *family-centered* ethics of medicine to replace the patient-centered ethics of traditional medicine and contemporary bioethics. From my perspective, a patient-centered ethics of medicine is morally perverse. A patient-centered bioethics cannot be justified when the rest of the family also has important interests at stake in treatment decisions—indeed, interests often more important than those of the patient. Families and loved ones must not be silenced. Families must not be reduced to "patient-support systems" or to means to the well-being of patients. We must, then, substitute a family-centered bioethics for a patient-centered bioethics. These are the themes that unite these essays.

I do not have a complete family-centered ethics to offer. In particular, I still lack adequate accounts of justice or fairness within a family, and also of how family decisions about medical treatment are to be made. I have not yet been able to write about many of the subtler features of family life. Still, each of these essays represents a journey toward a family-centered ethics of medicine beginning from a different starting point. They are united by the conviction that an ethics of health care must take seriously the fact that major illness is, indeed, "an illness in the family."

Most of the essays in this volume have been published previously and have not been revised for reprinting here. They are arranged in chronological order. Since all are variations on a theme, the reader is encouraged to read this volume selectively, beginning with the essay that looks most interesting and working out from there. Later essays in this volume do not require familiarity with earlier essays; in writing them, I could not assume an audience that would be familiar with my earlier work. Each essay had to stand by itself, and there is, unavoidably, considerable overlap and repetition among them.

The first essay—"In Search of an Ethics of Personal Relationships"—formulates my discomfort with the clumsy ways philosophers have talked about the ethics of personal relationships because of the impersonal context that philosophers tend to implicitly presuppose when they write about ethics. This essay will be of interest primarily to those concerned with philosophical ethics. "What About the Family?" is my first and most general statement of a family-centered bioethics. It provides perhaps the best general sketch of the project that unites this book. "The Problem of Proxies with Interests of Their Own" reflects on proxy decisions—decisions made on behalf of patients who cannot speak for themselves. Virtually all bioethicists subscribe to a theory of proxy decisions that is, I argue, badly mistaken. "SUPPORT and the Invisible Family" comments on one small piece of the famous and important SUPPORT study of medical treatment at the end of life. This part of the SUPPORT study, which documents the financial and lifestyle consequences for families resulting from decisions to extend the lives of very seriously ill and dying patients, has received little attention or comment. "Elder Abuse, Ethics, and Context" considers the problem of defining abuse in situations in which the family must provide extensive care for an ill or debilitated family member. Although this essay focuses on care of the elderly, there are important similarities in the analysis of the care—and the abuse—of younger family members. "Dying at the Right Time" discusses a good death and physician-assisted suicide from a perspective in which "a good death" includes more than simply what's best for the one who is dying. "Autobiography, Biography, and Narrative Ethics" addresses the central issue of who tells the story of an illness—who speaks, and who is silenced. To many, the entire line of thought I have been pursuing will seem to culminate in "Is There a Duty to Die?" A duty to die seems to carry a family-centered ethics all the way to the end of the line, to the most extreme conclusions that can be drawn from it.

A duty to die raises a host of troubling issues. My view that there is a fairly common duty to die is definitely a minority opinion, far from the prevailing wisdom of bioethics. Accordingly, I thought it important to include several different perspectives on this essay. Daniel Callahan, Larry Churchill, and Felicia Cohn and Joanne Lynn graciously agreed to comment on this essay. All have many other things they want to write, and I thank them. I have also reprinted Nat Hentoff's response from his widely syndicated column in *The Washington Post*. My final essay in this collection is a reply to these commentaries.

The afterword contains two sets of less abstractly theoretical reflections. The first is the personal responses of my own family to the essay, "Is There a Duty to Die?" One of the concerns raised by a duty to die is how it would affect the rest of the family. The responses of my family may not be representative, but my family has been living for several years with the awareness that one of their loved ones seriously believes he might one day have a duty to die. I thank my sons Bill and Jay, and my wife Mary for their reflections on an emotionally difficult subject. The second part of the afterword is a list of responsibilities of those facing the end of life. This list was formulated by a group of seniors, members of the Institute for Continued Learning in Johnson City, Tennessee. I thank them for permission to print this summary of their discussion. I think their list of responsibilities is an excellent starting point for discussion of the various dimensions of a responsible death.

I get by with a little help from my friends. I wish to thank Hilde and Jim Nelson, without whose assistance and advocacy this volume would not exist at all; Amelie Rorty for her support and encouragement at a critical point in my career; the physicians at the East Tennessee State University college of medicine who adopted a philosopher into their midst and patiently taught me something about medicine; my colleagues, mainly in the philosophy department at ETSU, who carefully read many earlier versions of these arguments; and especially my wife, Mary English, who helped me understand more about love, relationships, and family, and then worked with me to capture some of it in the words of these essays.

NOTES

1. The only book by bioethicists I know of that shows evidence of sustained reflection on families and health care is Nelson, Hilde L., and James L. Nelson, *The Patient in the Family*. New York: Routledge, 1995.

2. I have no definition of "family" to offer, but I do not restrict that notion to blood ties or legally sanctioned units. Although ties of blood and bonds of legality create their own set of issues, I am equally concerned about ties of affection and deep friendship. A deep, long-standing friendship is some patients' most important personal relationship; for some, it *is* their family. Nor do I assume that all family relationships are positive, supportive relationships. Ties of blood and marriage can create intensely antagonistic and hostile relationships. I believe that even the interests of a hateful and hostile family member are relevant to the ethics of treatment decisions, although the hostility is also a relevant factor. After all, hostility toward a relative does not make someone morally inconsiderable. Moreover, we dare not assume that the patient is innocent, that the hostility she now faces from her family is entirely unprovoked and unjustified.

In Search of an Ethics of Personal Relationships

Although it's been 10 years, I can still see the student, hands on her hips, as she brought my beautiful lecture on Kant's ethics to a grinding halt: "Is Kant saying," she demanded, "that if I sleep with my boyfriend, I should sleep with him out of a sense of duty?" My response: "And when you're through, you should tell him that you would have done the same for anyone in his situation." What could I say?

We do not search for what we already have. Thus my title commits me to the thesis that we do not yet have an ethics of personal relationships. And that is in fact my view, a view grown out of incidents like this one.

More specifically, I believe that for at least the past 300 years or so, philosophers thinking about ethics have tacitly presupposed a very impersonal context. They have unconsciously assumed a context in which we mean little or nothing to each other and have then asked themselves what principles could be invoked to keep us from trampling each other in the pursuit of our separate and often conflicting interests. Consequently, I contend, what we now study and teach under the rubric of ethics is almost entirely the ethics of impersonal relationships.

Various explanations might be offered as to why philosophers have thought in terms of impersonal relationships. Philosophers have historically been almost exclusively males, and males have generally believed that the public realm where impersonal relationships predominate is much more important and worthy of study than the private and personal dimensions of life. Or perhaps the assumption that we are talking about impersonal relationships reflects the growing impersonality of modern society or an awareness of the increasing ability given us by our technology to affect the lives of people quite remote from us.

However, even if philosophers were not thinking about personal relationships when developing their ethics, it might seem that an ethics adequate to impersonal relationships should work at least as well in personal contexts. For in personal relationships there would be less temptation to callously ignore or to ride roughshod over each other's interests, owing to the greater meaning each has for the other. Thus it seems reasonable to assume that the principles constituting the ethics of impersonal relationships will work satisfactorily in personal contexts as well.

But this assumption is false. An ethics of personal relationships must, I try to show, be quite different from the ethics of impersonal relationships. Traditional ethics is, at best, significantly incomplete, only a small part of the story of the ethics of personal relationships. Often it is much worse: basically misguided or wrong-headed and thus inapplicable in the context of personal relationships. In fact, much of traditional ethics urges us to act in ways that would be inappropriate in personal contexts; and thus traditional ethics would often be dangerous and destructive in those contexts.

We do not search for what we already have. I do not have an ethics of personal relationships, though I offer some suggestions about what such an ethics would and would *not* look like. Since my views about the ethics of personal relationships depend, naturally enough, on what I take a personal relationship to be, I begin with a brief discussion of the nature and structure of personal relationships.

But I'm going to cheat some: Throughout, I speak of personal relationships as if they were static. Although this is obviously a gross oversimplification, limitations of space and understanding preclude a discussion of the beginnings and endings and dynamics of personal relationships.

I

So what's a personal relationship? Personal relationships, as opposed to impersonal relationships, are of course relationships such as love, being lovers, friends, spouses, parents, and so on. But these sorts of relationships aren't always very *personal*, since there are all sorts of marriages of convenience, Aristotle's "friendships of utility,"

Hobbesian power alliances, and many varieties of quite impersonal sexual relationships. Consequently, we need to distinguish what are commonly *called* personal relationships (love, friendship, marriage) from personal relationships in a deeper sense. Even when they are not *personal* in the deeper sense, relationships like love, friendship, and marriage are not exactly impersonal relationships either. So I use the phrase "quasi-personal relationships" to cover such cases, reserving the term "personal relationships" for those relationships which are personal in the deeper sense I hope to explicate. I thus work with a threefold distinction between personal, quasi-personal, and impersonal relationships.

Let us begin with the distinction between personal and impersonal relationships. I want to say two things by way of characterizing personal relationships: (1) If I have a personal relationship with you, I want you. You (and your well-being) are then one of my *ends*. This would seem to be part of what it means to care for or care about another person. (2) If my relationship to you is to be personal, this end must be *you*—precisely you and not any other person. The persons in personal relationships are not substitutable, *salva affectione*.

Now, I need to explain these two points. But a full explanation of either would take at least a paper. And the first point raises all sorts of issues in action theory; the second, all sorts of metaphysical problems about what persons are and how they are individuated. Thus my strategy in this section is to say no more than necessary and to try to make that as susceptible to latitudinarian interpretation as possible. Hopefully, what I have to say will be acceptable to a broad spectrum of action theorists and metaphysicians. Ideally, all would be able to agree that there's something right and important about what I've said, and the familiar disputes could then be rejoined, including discussion of the presuppositions and implications of my statements.

First, then, the idea of having you as one of my ends is to be contrasted with both sides of the Kantian dichotomy between respecting you as an end in yourself and treating you as a means to my ends. Kant would have me respect you as a person, just as I would respect any person, simply because you (all) are persons. To respect you as an end in yourself is to recognize that you have value apart from whatever use I might be able to make of you. It is, moreover, to recognize that your goals and purposes have validity independent of whatever goals and purposes I may have and to acknowledge in my action that your goals and purposes have an equal claim to realization. Although respect for you and your goals is a part of a personal relationship, it is not what makes a personal relationship *personal*, valuable, or even a relationship. Instead, having you as one of my ends is valuing you in *relation* to me; it is seeing you and the realization of your goals as part of me and the realization of my goals. This is not, of course, to reduce you to a means to my ends. On the contrary, I want you. You are one of my *ends*.

The second characteristic of a personal relationship—that I want precisely *you*—serves to highlight the difference between this kind of relationship and impersonal relationships and also to further elucidate the difference between seeing you as one of my ends and seeing you either as an end in yourself or as a means to my ends. The characteristic intentions in personal relationships are different from those in impersonal relationships. It is the difference between:

wanting *to get* something (*T*) and wanting to get *T from you*.
wanting *to give* *T* and wanting to give *T to you*.
wanting *to do* *T* and wanting to do *T with you*.

The first set of intentions or desires structures impersonal relationships; the second, personal relationships. There is a big difference between wanting to be loved, for example, and wanting to be loved *by you*; a crucial difference between wanting to go to bed (with someone) and wanting to go to bed *with you*. This difference seems to retain its significance whether "*T*" ranges over relatively insignificant things like taking a walk, having your breakfast made, sharing a ride to a party, and going to a movie, or over crucially important things like baring your soul, receiving love and emotional support, sharing your living space, and having children.

If I want *something* (as opposed to wanting something *from you*), I depersonalize you, reducing you (in my eyes) to an *X* who is a possessor or producer of certain goods. For it's these good things I want, not you; anyone who could and would deliver these goods would do as well. The language captures the depersonalization nicely: I want "someone who. . . ." It is when I want *something* and you become for me a "someone who" is the possessor or producer of this good that I reduce you to a means to my ends. This kind of desire and the intentions it gives rise to structure an impersonal relationship, though many of what are usually called "personal relationships" are structured by precisely this sort of impersonal desire.

By contrast, in personal relationships of the deeper sort, "someone who. . . ." will not do; the specific person who is the object of my desire or intention cannot be substituted for or eliminated without altering the characteristic desire or intention. I see no way to explain how it could be important to me not only to receive some of the things I want, but to receive them *from you* unless we say that I see some sort of bond between you and me. I must value *you* over and above my valuing of whatever good things you are the possessor or producer of. The desire to receive *from you*/to give *to you*/to do *with you* thus structures a personal relationship, a relationship that does not reduce you to an *X* who is the bearer of goods and services. And this, it seems, is one clear sense of what it would mean to have *you* as one of my ends.

The possessiveness that often occurs in personal relationships can be seen to be closely analogous to the structure I have laid out here. If you are one of my ends, not only will I typically want your well-being, but I will also want to *create* your well-being. And if I want to give something personal to you, I will characteristically want you not only to receive it, but to receive it from me—not from just anyone. There may be nothing harmful in this, but it can easily slide into possessive jealousy. The structure of possessive jealousy seems to be this: I desire that *only* I give *T* to you/I want you to give *T only* to me/I want you to do *T only* with me. I can be said to be possessive with respect to all those *T*s, and jealousy will be aroused in me by the fear that these desires will not be fulfilled.

Let us now turn to quasi-personal relationships. These are the relationships that are commonly *called* personal, but that are not personal relationships in the deeper sense I have discussed. Quasi-personal relationships can be analyzed along similar lines. Suppose that it's important to me to have *the kind of friend* or *the kind of wife* who will help me with my work. In such cases, my desire or our relationship is not simply impersonal, for it won't do for me just to get help with my work—I want help from a friend or from a wife. In this intermediate case, the kind of relationship you have to me (wife, lover, loved one, friend, child) is essential to the structure of my desire; a certain kind of relationship is one of my ends.

But our relationship is still abstract or impersonal in a sense. I want something from you *because you are my wife* (lover, friend, child). I'd want the same from *any* wife (lover, friend, kid). Thus *you* are not important to the structure of my desire, *you* are not one of my ends. In such cases, the relationship I want must be defined (by me) in terms of roles and rules for those roles. I call these relationships quasi-personal. They are important for an ethics of personal relationships, for we often get hurt in precisely these sorts of relationships, especially when we believe we are involved in a personal relationship.

Two additional points about personal relationships are important for the ethics of personal relationships. First, although I talk mainly about positive, healthy personal relationships, it is important to recognize that *hatred*, as well as love, can be a personal relationship. As can resentment, anger, contempt. Hatred is personal if I hate *you*, not just some of the things you are or do or stand for, not just "anyone who. . . ." In cases of personal hatred, I may well desire your overall ill-being. Hatred that is personal rather than impersonal is much more thoroughgoing and often more vicious. Good sense suggests that we should get out of or depersonalize relationships dominated by intractable hatred, anger, or resentment. Interestingly, however, haters often don't get out of personal relationships with those they hate. And this calls for explanation. Such explanation must acknowledge that if I continue to hate *you* and to have your ill-being as one of my ends, there must be some sort of bond between you and me. *You* are important to me or I wouldn't devote my life to making *you* miserable. The opposite of love is not hatred; the opposite of love is indifference.

A second point important for the ethics of personal relationships is the possibility of one-sided personal relationships. Suppose I want *you* and you simply want to be loved and protected or to have a certain kind of marriage. Do I then have a personal relationship with you while you have an impersonal or quasi-personal relationship with me? Perhaps. But this surely is not the kind of relationship I will normally want. Such relationships are ripe for exploitation and tragedy. They are, in any case, almost always deeply disappointing, for we usually want *mutually* personal relationships. This means that not only do I want *you* and not just some producer of certain goods and services, but I want you to want *me*, not "someone who. . . ."

Although the logical structure of personal, quasi-personal, and impersonal relationships seems quite distinct, there can be tremendous epistemic difficulties facing those of us who would know what kinds of relationships we have. Do I want *you* or do I want *something* (from you)? Do I want a relationship *with you* or do I want a *kind* of relationship with "someone who. . ."? Even if I think I want you, is it because I'm picking up on something that is *you*, or is it because you happen to resemble my childhood sweetheart, perhaps, or because you are so successful? If I cannot fathom my desires and intentions enough to make these discriminations accurately, it would be possible for me not to know whether I have a personal relationship with you, much less whether you have a personal relationship with me. These epistemic difficulties notwithstanding, it may be *critically* important—both ethically and psychologically—to know what kinds of relationships we actually do have. Relationships are often made or broken by the issue of whether I want you or "someone who. . . ."

Despite the distinct logical structures, it's probably also true that most of what are usually called "personal relationships" contain elements of all three—impersonal, quasi-personal, and personal relationships. (In fact, the best personal relationships may contain elements of the impersonal in them: Clearly, it is crucial to a healthy relationship that I not want to get *from you* everything that I want. You would be smothered by endless demands in such a relationship.) Nonetheless, we can sort actual relationships into these three types if we can talk about the dominant or characteristic kind of intention involved in a given relationship. Or if we consider personal and impersonal relationships to be ideal types marking the ends of a spectrum, the points along this spectrum will be determined by how centrally personal desires and intentions figure in various relationships.

Obviously, these characterizations of personal and quasi-personal relationships are based on my own intuitions, with which others may not agree. Fortunately, my argument does not require that my characterizations be accepted as necessary conditions, much less as necessary and sufficient conditions, for a personal relationship. It is enough for my purposes if it is admitted that many very healthy and beautiful personal relationships have the structure I have ascribed to them and that the reasons we often have for wanting personal relationships are expressed in my formulations.

II

Now for the ethics of personal relationships. My main contention and basic principle is that ethics must not depersonalize personal relationships, for doing so does violence to what these relationship are; to what is characteristically and normatively going on in them; and to the intentions, desires, and hopes we have in becoming involved in them. Particular persons figure essentially in personal relationships. But most ways of thinking about ethics invite or require us to treat ourselves or our loved ones as a "someone who. . . ." And this leads to many difficulties, both on the level of metaethical theory and on the practical level of ethical or moral prescription.

Some of the points I want to draw attention to have already been made by Michael Stocker (1976) and Bernard Williams (1976). But they bear repetition in this context. It is instructive that both Stocker and Williams turn to examples of personal relationships to illustrate their points. Though both want to make general points about ethical theory, I would contend that many of their points are plausible and defensible only or primarily in the context of personal relationships.

The main thrust of this section of the paper is critical, outlining some of the ways in which most approaches to ethics are not appropriate to personal relationships. The next section offers more positive suggestions about what an ethics and metaethics of personal relationships would have to look like. Obviously, it goes without saying that in a paper that proposes to reject all major ethical traditions and then to suggest an alternative to them, none of the arguments can be conclusive. I can hope only to point toward a different perspective, inviting you to examine your experience and your sense of personal relationships to see whether there is anything in what I have to say.

Kantian ethics depersonalizes all personal relationships. Since Kant generally recognizes no community except the kingdom of ends, he leaves us with the false dichotomy either of choosing to pursue our own atomistic goals and reducing others to a means thereto or of promoting the kingdom of ends in which we respect others because they are instances of moral agency. In other words, Kant fails to recognize that, in addition to being a means to my ends or an end in yourself, you can be one of *my ends*.

It is personal affirmation that one wants from a personal relationship, not respect as a moral agent or even respect or admiration for one's nonmoral qualities. Thus respect of a kind that is due to *anyone* is not sufficient to generate an ethics of personal relationships. Nor can such an ethics be generated by adding consideration of the special obligations generated by the *kind* of relationships we stand in—lovers, friends, spouses, or whatever. Rather, desiring a mutually personal relationship, I want you to want *me*, not "someone who. . . ." I certainly do not want you to want me simply because I am a moral agent, or even primarily because I am a responsible moral agent.

The difficulties extend beyond Kantian ethics. Any ethics that is formulated in terms of what "*one* would have done for *anyone* in a certain kind of situation" or that talks as if there could be moral situations involving different agents that are "the same in all morally relevant respects" depersonalizes personal relationships. Thus if rights, duties, and obligations must be impersonally or quasi-personally defined—as I think they must be—they depersonalize relationships, reducing those involved in the relationships to a "someone who. . . ."

The concept of a rule is so very general that I hesitate to say that no rules are applicable in personal relationships. But I would claim that no set of general rules or principles will adequately describe personal interaction (in the deeper sense) or adequately prescribe an ethics of personal relationships. The ethics of personal relationships will not be primarily an ethics of rules. And the rules or norms there are must be contextually defined; instead of striving to achieve a universally valid viewpoint, one strives to understand and be moved by the particular point of view of the specific other. And one hopes for the same understanding in return.

Moreover, even if it should turn out that rules *are* an essential component of the ethics of personal relationships, they will standardly be different from the rules that apply in impersonal contexts. If we are close and I know that you care for me and will keep my interest in mind, you don't have to obey the rules for impersonal relationships. You can, for example, invade my privacy by cross-examining me about my personal life, disrupt what I'm doing for no better reason than that you're at loose ends and want someone to talk to, or fail to respect my private property by taking $20 from my wallet, removing a book from my office, or borrowing my car without permission. All that is fine, so long as I am convinced that you care for me.

In fact, it would be insulting or deeply troubling (if not ludicrous) if you *did* obey the rules for impersonal relationships, for freedom from those rules is one of the signs by which we show that we appreciate that the relationship is personal. Imagine finding out that a close friend has been depressed for some time and has wanted to talk with you, but hasn't called because he didn't want to interrupt what you were doing. Or imagine returning from a summer in Europe to find that a friend had been seriously hampered in her attempt to write a paper because she didn't feel free to take a copy of a book she knew you had in your office.

Because act utilitarianism is not an ethics of rules, it seems closer to the mark than rule utilitarianism. But both forms of utilitarianism tend to reduce personal relationships to a means to more ultimate goods—happiness, for example. Nor will it do simply to include friendship or love as one part of the good, for that is still a *kind* of relationship, not *our* relationship. This distinction is not trivial or academic: Consider how it would feel to discover that your loved one just wanted love, not you or your relationship.

Moreover, because an impersonal ethics like utilitarianism or Kantianism asks us to abstract from consideration of our particular relationships, it generates an impartiality that makes it difficult for us to justify our decisions within personal relationships. And even if it can justify those decisions, its way of doing so would depersonalize us, our partners, and our relationships. Suppose that as she climbed into bed, my wife told me that she'd faced a difficult moral decision about coming home to sleep with me because there were many men who were much more lonely and who would have benefited so much more than I, if she'd slept with them, instead. However (she continued), on utilitarian grounds she decided that the institutions of love and marriage produce more happiness than alternative arrangements, so she decided it was right to come home in order to support those institutions. Wouldn't that be splendid!

Contract theories (Hobbes, Locke, Rawls) don't fare much better; it is not clear that they can be extended beyond the impersonal contexts for which they were formulated and in which they are at home. Indeed, the whole point of contract theory is to try to get us to abstract from our particular characteristics, wants, goals, and values, in order to ascertain what any self-interested, rational being would want and, given those wants, would agree to. Not surprisingly, such depersonalized contractors agree only to principles for impersonal and quasi-personal relationships. Stripped of all particular characteristics, it is impossible to tell whether you'd want personal relationships at all (some people do not), though it might be prudent to make allowances just in case you did. Stripped of all particular characteristics, it is clearly impossible to tell whether you would want *me* and *our* relationship. Only impersonal and quasi-personal relationships are visible behind the veil of ignorance.

There is an even deeper difficulty. Contract theory asks us to see ourselves as atoms. If I see myself as an atom, I see my own well-being as separate from the well-being of others—separate, to be sure, not in the sense that there are no causal relationships between my well-being and that of others, but in the sense that I do not see their well-being as *part* of mine. Those who see themselves as atoms are not necessarily selfish or immoral—they can be impartial, benevolent, even generous in their actions. But they bestow benefits as they receive them—on "someone who's" who are not essentially related to their own well-being.

Contract theory thus tacitly reduces all relationship between us to trade relationships. And trade relationships cannot provide an adequate model for personal relationships. If I do not see *you* as part of me and my well-being, I do not want *you*. I can only want *something* from you. And if I only want *something*, as opposed to wanting something *from you*, for me you are only a means to my well-being. If you (also seeing yourself as an atom) also only want something, ours becomes what I call a "trade relationship." This is true, even if we trade very intimate and personal things like sex, companionship, emotional support. Even love (or a reasonable facsimile thereof) can be traded—if we both want love, not each other. Then we use each other and we become means to each other's ends.

Finally, consider an Aristotelian ethics of virtue. An ethics of virtue may be closer to meeting the requirements of an ethics of personal relationships. But the fact that the girl next door is virtuous does not ensure that she will be a good friend, much less a good friend *to me*. Virtue theory also threatens to depersonalize persons— a good person is a kind of person, a "someone who. . . ." And thus virtue theory may also miss the *personal* attraction and affirmation that are the core of personal relationships. (Remember when your mother or father used to tell you that you should be interested in someone because he or she is "such a good person"?)

This is not, of course, to say that good relationships are possible with those totally devoid of virtues. But even if virtue theory would give us the kind of metaethics we want, the ethics of impersonal relationships will still be critically different from the ethics of personal relationships. For the virtues required in personal relationships are different from those required in impersonal contexts. They may, in fact, not even be wholly compatible with the impersonal virtues.

Consider, for example, impartiality and impartial justice, which are a virtue in an employer, but a vice in a father, mother, or spouse. Thus the dilemma posed by nepotism: qua employer one should treat all applicants impartially, but qua parent one is defective if one is not willing to provide special advantages to one's children. I believe closer examination would reveal that even those virtues that seem applicable in both personal and impersonal contexts—care, honesty, fairness—have different meanings in personal and impersonal contexts. Compare the care of one who devotes a lifetime to the work of Oxfam with the care of a mother for her child.

In addition, insofar as virtue theory specifies virtues in terms of social practices that must be defined by a society larger than a couple, development of the requisite virtues could yield only a quasi-personal relationship—a *kind* of relationship, at best. And the personal affirmation we desire from marriage, for example, would be missing in a virtuous husband or wife as much as it would in a Kantian universalizer, a utilitarian calculator, or a rational contractor.

Thus all our major traditions in ethics strike me as inadequate to an ethics of personal relationships. And inadequate not simply by virtue of incompleteness. Rather, they seem fundamentally wrong-headed. Granted, someone ingenious enough might be able to devise a system of epicycles that would harmonize existing ethical theories with the ethics of personal relationships. But my own sense is that the errors lie much deeper and that something basically different is required.

III

"I don't want you to take me out," my wife exploded. "I just want you to want to go out with me. If you don't want to go out, let's just forget it." Motives, intentions, and reasons for acting play a *much* larger role in the ethics of personal relationships than they do in the ethics of impersonal relationships. In fact, the motivation of those who are close to us is often more important than the things which result from it. And even when actions are important in personal relationships, it is often because they are seen as symbols or symptoms of underlying feelings, desires, or commitments. Thus actions often seem worthless or even perverse if the motivation behind them is inappropriate.

In impersonal situations and relationships, on the other hand, we are much more content to allow people to do the right thing for the wrong reason, and we are often even willing to provide incentives (for example, legal and financial) to increase the chances that they will do the right thing and also that they will do it for the wrong reason. I wouldn't, for example, be very much concerned about the motives of my congressman if I could be sure that he would always vote right. I believe that he should be well paid to increase the chances that he will vote right. But I would be deeply upset to learn that my wife is staying with me primarily for financial reasons. And I might be even more upset if her actions all along had been scrupulously wifelike. An ethics of personal relationships must, then, place more emphasis on motives and intentions, less on actions and consequences than most ethical theories have.

However, the motives that ethicists have found praiseworthy in impersonal contexts are usually inappropriate and unacceptable in personal contexts. Actions motivated by duty, a sense of obligation, or even a sense of responsibility are often unacceptable in personal relationships. A healthy personal relationship cannot be based on this sort of motivation; indeed, it cannot even come into play very often. Stocker's example of learning that your friend has come to see you in the hospital purely from a sense of duty is telling. Even more devastating would be to learn that your spouse of 37 years had stayed in your marriage purely or even primarily out of a sense of obligation stemming from the marriage contract.

For similar reasons, motives of benevolence, pity, or compassion are also not acceptable as the characteristic or dominant motives in personal relationships. Acts of charity, altruism, and mercy are also, in general, out. As are sacrifices of important interests or a sense of self-sacrifice. Paternalism and maternalism are also generally unacceptable among adults in personal relationships. While it might be nice to feel yourself to be charitable, benevolent, or compassionate, who could endure being emotionally involved with someone who saw you essentially or even very often as an appropriate object of benevolence, charity, or pity? Of course, there always will be some occasions when you *are* an appropriate object of these attitudes, and it's desirable that they then be forthcoming . . . so long as they are viewed as exceptions. And yet, even in cases of great misfortune—if I contracted a debilitating disease, for example—I don't think I'd want my wife or friends to stay with me if they were motivated predominantly by pity or benevolence.

If even this much is correct, I think we can draw several lessons that point toward a deeper understanding of ethics in personal relationships. First, personal relationships between adults (and perhaps also between adults and children) are to be entered into and continued out of a sense of strength, fullness, and vitality, both in yourself and in the other, not out of a sense of weakness, need, emptiness, or incapacity.

Anything other than a shared sense of vitality and strength would lead to the unacceptable motives already discussed. Moreover, if I see myself primarily as a being in need, I will be too focused on myself and my needs. I will then tend to depersonalize you into a someone who can meet my needs. And I will also be generally unable to freely and joyously give: Since I see myself as not having enough as it is, my giving will seem to me a giving up. (Does this mean that those who most need a first-rate personal relationship will be unable to have one? I'm afraid that this might be true.)

The fact that giving characteristically must be free and joyous points to a second lesson about the ethics of personal relationships: Characteristically and normatively, the appropriate motive for action in personal relationships is simply that we want to do these things. Persons pursue whatever *ends* they have simply because they want to (that's what it means to say that something is an *end*, of course). And in a personal relationship, I and my well-being are ends of yours. From this vantage point it is easy to see why motives should play such a central role in personal relationships and also why *wanting* to do the things we do together is often the only acceptable motivation: That motivation is the touchstone of whether or not we have a personal relationship.

Of course, this is not to imply that personal relationships must rest simply on untutored feelings, taken as brute givens in the personalities of the participants. Indeed, it makes sense to talk about doing things, even for the wrong reasons, in order that doing those things will in time change you, your feelings, and your reasons. But it may be even more important to point out that continual attempts to create the right feelings in oneself are also not acceptable or satisfactory. If you must continually try to get yourself to want to do things with me, or for me, or for our relationship, we must at some point admit that I and my well-being are not among your ends and that we do not, therefore, have a personal relationship.

Nor am I claiming that actions motivated by a sense of duty or obligation, by altruism or self-sacrifice, by benevolence, pity, charity, sympathy, and so on *never* have a place in personal relationships. They may be appropriate in unusual circumstances. But such motives and actions are a fall-back mechanism which I compare to the safety net beneath a high-wire act. We may be safer with a net, but the act is no good if the net actually comes into play very often. Similarly, the fallback mechanisms may, in times of crisis, protect us and *some* of what we want, but they do not and cannot safeguard what is central to personal relationships. Thus when we find ourselves thinking characteristically or even very often in terms of the motives and concepts I have claimed are generally inappropriate in personal relationships, this is a symptom that our relationships are unsound, unhealthy, jeopardized, decayed, or that they never did become the personal relationships we wanted and hoped for. (Compare Hardwig, 1984.)

A third lesson about the ethics of personal relationships can be drawn from these reflections: The distinction between egoism and altruism is not characteristically applicable to personal relationships. Neither party magnanimously or ignominiously sacrifices personal interests, but the two interests are not independent, not really even two. For your ends are my ends too. The distinction between giving and receiving thus collapses. In impersonal contexts, if I respect your (independent) interests, that may be all you want of me. But in a personal context, you will want me to be interested in your interests. For if I am not interested in your interests, your well-being is not one of my ends.

This does not, of course, mean that all interests will be shared, but it means I am interested even in those of your interests I do not share. (I may have no appreciation of operas, but knowing how much they mean to you, it is important to me that your life include them. Operas for you are important to me in a way that operas for others who may love them just as much simply are not.) Nor, of course, am I claiming that there are *never* conflicts of interest in personal relationships. But such conflicts are set within the context of the meaning each has for the other and are therefore seen and handled differently. In personal relationships, conflicts of interest are conflicts within myself, a very different thing from a conflict of interest with someone separate from me.

A fourth lesson about ethics and personal relationships is this: Because personal relationships are ends—indeed, ultimate and incommensurable ends—they cannot and need not be justified by an appeal to some higher value such as love, pleasure, utility, or social utility. Any ethics that attempts to justify personal relationships in terms of more ultimate goods depersonalizes personal relationships. It construes us as wanting these higher goods, not each other.

Nor can the relative merits of personal relationships be adequately assessed in terms of abstract values. Each personal relationship is a good *sui generis*. Irreducibly involving the specific persons that they do, personal relationships cannot be reduced to common denominators that would permit comparison without depersonalizing them. Although persons caught in situations requiring choices between different personal relationships sometimes talk (and probably think) about comparing them in terms of abstract common denominators, evaluating relationships in this way Platonistically reduces our loved ones to mere instantiations of forms, thus depersonalizing them and our relationships to them.

A fifth and final lesson serves to summarize and conclude these reflections. The ethics of personal relationships must see persons in nonatomic terms; it must be based on a doctrine of internal relations. People see themselves in nonatomic terms if they see at least some other individuals not just as means to their well-being, but as part of their well-being. As I suggested earlier, there is no way to explain why I value a relationship with *you* (over and above the goods I desire from you and from this kind of relationship) except by saying that I feel a bond between us. I have come to see myself as a self that can only be fulfilled by a life that includes a relationship with you. Thus I see myself, in part, as part of a larger whole that is *us*. This does not mean that I see you as either a necessary or a sufficient condition for my well-being. If our relationship ends, my world will not fall apart and I may know that it won't. But if our relationship does end, I will have to alter my conception of myself and my well-being.

IV

Those wedded to the traditional categories of ethics could accept most of the points I have wanted to make and yet insist that what I have called the ethics of personal relationships cannot be an *ethics*, since it does not meet the criteria that define the moral point of view. Even if correct, my observations about appropriate conduct in personal relationships would, on that view, be applied psychology perhaps, or some sort of prudential reasoning about how to have better relationships. But I would claim that such a reaction would only show the extent to which we have unknowingly accepted an ethics appropriate to impersonal contexts as definitive of all ethics.

Others might object that a position such as mine faces an insuperable dilemma: Either ethics is unnecessary in personal relationships or the kind of ethics I have been advocating will not work. On this view, ethics is unnecessary where genuine care is present in a personal relationship, since we don't need an ethics to protect us from those who understand us and care about our interests. But, it might be claimed, in unhealthy or destructive personal relationship—or even relationships that are temporarily strained—what I have been calling the ethics of personal relationships simply will not work. The conclusion of this argument would be that we need an ethics of rules and principles, rights and duties whenever real caring is absent or even obscured—especially, perhaps, in personal relationships, where anger, hatred, bitterness, and resentment are often so thoroughgoing, intractable, and . . . personal.

Granted, we must remember that relationships can be viciously personal as well as gloriously personal. And it does seem plausible to maintain that we don't need an ethics for times when relationships are healthy and going smoothly. But again, I believe that the plausibility of this view reflects the limitations of the ways in which we have thought about ethics. I would contend, instead, that we *do* need an ethics for good times and for healthy, beautiful relationship—an ethics of *aspiration* that would serve to clarify what we aim for in personal relationships and to remind us of how they are best done.

Moreover, even when personal relationships become troubled, strained, or even vicious, it is not always possible or desirable to depersonalize the relationship. And an ethics must not tacitly urge or require us to depersonalize our relationships whenever serious conflicts arise. Within a personal relationship, the depersonalizing stance will often distort the issue beyond recognition. If we leave out my love for you, my turmoil over how often you drink yourself into oblivion vanishes, and with it, the issue that arises between us. For I can acknowledge with equanimity the drinking of others who are not personally related to me. My concern is simply not an impersonal concern that ranges indifferently over many possible objects of concern.

Depersonalizing (or ending) a relationship *may* be the appropriate final step in the face of intractable difficulties. But I would deny that depersonalizing is always the best course even here. For I think we should aspire to learn how to end relationships without depersonalizing them. If we can learn to continue to care and to care personally for our past loves, friends, and partners, we can be left happier, less bitter, wiser about the causes of the difficulties, and better able to go on to other relationships than if we end our relationships in hostility, anger, rejection, or even the kind of indifference characteristic of an impersonal stance.

What, then, is to be done? If we accept my position that we need an ethics of personal relationships and that such an ethics will have to be different from an ethics of impersonal relationships, the field of ethics opens up and ethical theory turns out to be a much less thoroughly explored domain than we might have thought. For my view implies that there are vast, largely uncharted regions beyond what we have come to know as ethics. I have tried to point to this region, but I have hardly begun to explore it.

1. We need to consider whether personal relationships are always better. If that view is correct, impersonal relationships would be only the result of the limitations of our sense of relatedness, and there would be a constant ethical imperative to personalize social contexts whenever possible and to expand our sense of connectedness. I suspect, however, that some relationships are better left impersonal and also that, because enmity, resentment, disgust, and many forms of conflict are much more bitter and intractable when they are personal, there are situations where depersonalizing is a good strategy. We must also understand more clearly exactly what depersonalizing a relationship involves.

2. We need an ethics for quasi-personal relationships (love, marriage, friendship) when these relationships are not also personal (in the sense I have been trying to explicate). For it is perhaps in such contexts that people are most devastatingly used, abused, and mistreated. Still, quasi-personal relationships have important roles to play, both when they do and when they do not involve a personal relationship: Marriage is also a financial institution; our concept of a parent seeks to ensure that children will be protected and raised, even if not loved; even living together is in part an arrangement for sharing the chores of daily life.

3. We need some way to deal with the conflicts and tensions arising in situations involving both personal and impersonal relationships. Is it moral, for example, for me to buy computer games and gold chains for my son while other children are starving, simply because he is my son and I have a personal relationship with him? The issues about the extent to which one can legitimately favor those to whom one is personally related are, for me, deeply troubling and almost impenetrable to my ethical insight. On the more theoretical level, we can see the difficulties that those committed to impersonal

value—such as consequentialists and Kantians—have with personal commitments, and also the difficulties that feminist ethicists—such as Gilligan (1982) and Noddings (1984) have with conduct toward those not part of our network of care as conflicts arise between the demands of personal and of impersonal ethics.

4. Then, when we have all this in view, we should perhaps reexamine our "stranger ethics" to see if we need to revise our ethics of impersonal relationships in light of the ethics of personal and quasi-personal relationships.

5. Finally, we undoubtedly need a more precise understanding of what makes relationships personal, a better grasp on the values of such relationships, and a much more rigorous and developed account of the ethics of personal relationships. For even if the present paper succeeds beyond my wildest dreams, it has only scratched the surface.

Until we have done all these things, it will be premature to make pronouncements about what constitutes "the moral point of view."

ACKNOWLEDGMENTS

This paper was begun in 1978 at a National Endowment for the Humanities Summer Seminar directed by Amelie Rorty. It has, in various versions, benefited from many helpful criticisms and suggestions from the members of that NEH seminar, from the Philosophy Departments at East Tennessee State University and Virginia Commonwealth University, from the members of Kathy Emmett's seminar on personal relationships, from the editors of the present volume, and especially from Amelie Rorty and Mary Read English. My many benefactors have left me with a whole sheaf of powerful and important ideas for revising, amending, and qualifying what I've said, but unfortunately too often without the wit and wisdom needed to incorporate their suggestions into this paper.

REFERENCES

Gilligan, C. *In a Different Voice: Psychological Theory and Women's Development*. Cambridge: Harvard University Press, 1982.

Hardwig, J. "Should Women Think in Terms of Rights?" *Ethics*, 94 (1984): 441–55.
Noddings, N. *Caring: A Feminine Approach to Ethics and Moral Education*. Berkeley: University of California Press, 1984.

Stocker, M. "The Schizophrenia of Modern Ethical Theories." *Journal of Philosophy*, 73 (1976): 453–66.

Williams, B. "Persons, Character, and Morality." *The Identities of Persons*. Ed. A. G. Rorty. Berkeley: University of California Press, 1976.

What About the Family?

We are beginning to recognize that the prevalent ethic of patient autonomy simply will not do. Since demands for health care are virtually unlimited, giving autonomous patients the care they want will bankrupt our health care system. We can no longer simply buy our way out of difficult questions of justice by expanding the health care pie until there is enough to satisfy the wants and needs of everyone. The requirements of justice and the needs of other patients must temper the claims of autonomous patients.

But if the legitimate claims of other patients and other (nonmedical) interests of society are beginning to be recognized, another question is still largely ignored: To what extent can the patient's family legitimately be asked or required to sacrifice their interests so that the patient can have the treatment he or she wants?

This question is not only almost universally ignored, it is generally implicitly dismissed, silenced before it can even be raised. This tacit dismissal results from a fundamental assumption of medical ethics: Medical treatment ought always to serve the interests of the patient. This, of course, implies that the interests of family members should be irrelevant to medical treatment decisions or at least ought never to take precedence over the interests of the patient. All questions about fairness to the interests of family members are thus precluded, regardless of the merit or importance of the interests that will have to be sacrificed if the patient is to receive optimal treatment.

Yet there is a whole range of cases in which important interests of family members are dramatically affected by decisions about the patient's treatment; medical decisions often should be made with those interests in mind. Indeed, in many cases family members have a greater interest than the patient in which treatment option is exercised. In such cases, the interests of family members often ought to *override* those of the patient.

The problem of family interests cannot be resolved by considering other members of the family as "patients," thereby redefining the problem as one of conflicting interests among *patients*. Other members of the family are not always ill, and even if ill, they still may not be patients. Nor will it do to define the whole family as one patient. Granted, the slogan "the patient is the family" was coined partly to draw attention to precisely the issues I wish to raise, but the idea that the whole family is one patient is too monolithic. The conflicts of interests, beliefs, and values among family members are often too real and run too deep to treat all members as "the patient." Thus, if I am correct, it is sometimes the moral thing to do for a physician to sacrifice the interests of her patient to those of nonpatients—specifically, to those of the other members of the patient's family.

But what is the "family"? As I will use it here, it will mean roughly "those who are close to the patient." "Family" so defined will often include close friends and companions. It may also exclude some with blood or marriage ties to the patient. "Closeness" does not, however, always mean care and abiding affection, nor need it be a positive experience—one can hate, resent, fear, or despise a mother or brother with an intensity not often directed toward strangers, acquaintances, or associates. But there are cases where even a hateful or resentful family member's interests ought to be considered.

This use of "family" gives rise to very sensitive ethical—and legal—issues in the case of legal relatives with no emotional ties to the patient that I cannot pursue here. I can only say that I do not mean to suggest that the interests of legal relatives who are not emotionally close to the patient are always to be ignored. They will sometimes have an important financial interest in the treatment even if they are not emotionally close to the patient. But blood and marriage ties can become so thin that they become *merely* legal relationships. (Consider, for example, "couples" who have long since parted but who have never gotten a divorce, or cases in which the next of kin cannot be bothered with making proxy decisions.) Obviously, there are many important questions about just whose interests are to be considered in which treatment decisions and to what extent.

CONNECTED INTERESTS

There is no way to detach the lives of patients from the lives of those who are close to them. Indeed, the intertwining of lives is part of the very meaning of closeness. Consequently, there will be a broad spectrum of cases in which the treatment options will have dramatic and different impacts on the patient's family.

I believe there are many, many such cases. To save the life of a newborn with serious defects is often dramatically to affect the rest of the parents' lives and, if they have other children, may seriously compromise the quality of their lives, as well. . . . The husband of a woman with Alzheimer's disease may well have a life totally dominated for 10 years or more by caring for an increasingly foreign and estranged wife. . . . The choice between aggressive and palliative care or, for that matter, the difference between either kind of care and suicide in the case of a father with terminal cancer or AIDS may have a dramatic emotional and financial impact on his wife and children. . . . Less dramatically, the choice between two medications, one of which has the side effect of impotence, may radically alter the life a couple has together. . . . The drug of choice for controlling high blood pressure may be too expensive (that is, requires too many sacrifices) for many families with incomes just above the ceiling for Medicaid. . . .

Because the lives of those who are close are not separable, to be close is to no longer have a life entirely your own to live entirely as you choose. To be part of a family is to be morally required to make decisions on the basis of thinking about what is best for all concerned, not simply what is best for yourself. In healthy families, characterized by genuine care, one wants to make decisions on this basis, and many people do so quite naturally and automatically. My own grandfather committed suicide after his heart attack as a final gift to his wife—he had plenty of life insurance but not nearly enough health insurance, and he feared that she would be left homeless and destitute if he lingered on in an incapacitated state. Even if one is not so inclined, however, it is irresponsible and wrong to exclude or to fail to consider the interests of those who are close. Only when the lives of family members will not be importantly affected can one rightly make exclusively or even predominantly self-regarding decisions.

Although "what is best for all concerned" sounds utilitarian, my position does not imply that the right course of action results simply from a calculation of what is best for all. No, the seriously ill may have a right to special consideration, and the family of an ill person may have a duty to make sacrifices to respond to a member's illness. It is one thing to claim that the ill deserve special consideration; it is quite another to maintain that they deserve exclusive or even over-riding consideration. Surely we must admit that there are limits to the right to special treatment by virtue of illness. Otherwise, everyone would be morally required to sacrifice all other goods to better care for the ill. We must also recognize that patients too have moral oblig-ations, obligations to try to protect the lives of their families from destruction resulting from their illnesses.

Thus, unless serious illness excuses one from all moral respon-sibility—and I don't see how it could—it is an oversimplification to say of a patient who is part of a family that "it's his life" or "after all, it's his medical treatment," as if his life and his treatment could be successfully isolated from the lives of the other members of his fami-ly. It is more accurate to say "it's their lives" or "after all, they're all going to have to live with his treatment." Then the really serious moral questions are not *whether* the interests of family members are relevant to decisions about a patient's medical treatment or *whether* their interests should be included in his deliberations or in delibera-tions about him, but how far family and friends can be asked to sup-port and sustain the patient. What sacrifices can they be morally required to make for his health care? How far can they reasonably be asked to compromise the quality of their lives so that he will receive the care that would improve the quality of his life? To what extent can he reasonably expect them to put their lives "on hold" to preoc-cupy themselves with his illness to the extent necessary to care for him?

THE ANOMALY OF MEDICAL DECISION MAKING

The way we analyze medical treatment decisions by or for patients is plainly anomalous to the way we think about other important deci-sions family members make. I am a husband, a father, and still a son, and no one would argue that I should or even responsibly could decide to take a sabbatical, another job, or even a weekend trip *solely* on the basis of what I want for myself. Why should decisions about my medical treatment be different? Why should we have even *thought* that medical treatment decisions might be different?

Is it because medical decisions, uniquely, involve life and death matters? Most medical decisions, however, are not matters of life and death, and we as a society risk or shorten the lives of other people—through our toxic waste disposal decisions, for example—quite apart from considerations of whether that is what they want for themselves.

Have we been misled by a preoccupation with the biophysical model of disease? Perhaps it has tempted us to think of illness and hence also of treatment as something that takes place *within* the body of the patient. What happens in my body does not—barring contagion—affect my wife's body, yet it usually does affect her.

Have we tacitly desired to simplify the practice and the ethics of medicine by considering only the *medical* or health-related consequences of treatment decisions? Perhaps, but it is obvious that we need a broader vision of and sensitivity to *all* the consequences of action, at least among those who are not simply technicians following orders from above. Generals need to consider more than military consequences, businessmen more than economic consequences, teachers more than educational consequences, lawyers more than legal consequences.

Does the weakness and vulnerability of serious illness imply that the ill need such protection that we should serve only their interests? Those who are sick may indeed need special protection, but this can only mean that we must take special care to see that the interests of the ill are duly considered. It does not follow that their interests are to be served exclusively or even that their interests must always predominate. Moreover, we must remember that in terms of the dynamics of the family, the patient is not always the weakest member, the member most in need of protection.

Does it make *historical*, if not logical, sense to view the wishes and interests of the patient as always overriding? Historically, illnesses were generally of much shorter duration; patients got better quickly or died quickly. Moreover, the costs of the medical care available were small enough that rarely was one's future mortgaged to the costs of the care of family members. Although this was once truer than it is today, there have always been significant exceptions to these generalizations.

None of these considerations adequately explains why the interests of the patient's family have been thought to be appropriately excluded from consideration. At the very least, those who believe that medical treatment decisions are morally anomalous to other important decisions owe us a better account of how and why this is so.

LIMITS OF PUBLIC POLICY

It might be thought that the problem of family interests *is* a problem only because our society does not shelter families from the negative effects of medical decisions. If, for example, we adopted a comprehensive system of national health insurance and also a system of public insurance to guarantee the incomes of families, then my sons' chances at a college education and the quality of the rest of their lives might not have to be sacrificed were I to receive optimal medical care.

However, it is worth pointing out that we are still moving primarily in the *opposite* direction. Instead of designing policies that would increasingly shelter family members from the adverse impact of serious and prolonged illnesses, we are still attempting to shift the burden of care to family members in our efforts to contain medical costs. A social system that would safeguard families from the impact of serious illness is nowhere in sight in this country. And we must not do medical ethics as if it were.

It is perhaps even more important to recognize that the lives of family members could not be sheltered from all the important ramifications of medical treatment decisions by *any* set of public policies. In any society in which people get close to each other and care deeply for each other, treatment decisions about one will often and *irremediably* affect more than one. If a newborn has been saved by aggressive treatment but is severely handicapped, the parents may simply not be emotionally capable of abandoning the child to institutional care. A man whose wife is suffering from multiple sclerosis may simply not be willing or able to go on with his own life until he sees her through to the end. A woman whose husband is being maintained in a vegetative state may not feel free to marry or even to see other men again, regardless of what some revised law might say about her marital status.

Nor could we desire a society in which friends and family would quickly lose their concern as soon as continuing to care began to diminish the quality of their own lives. For we would then have alliances for better but not for worse, in health but not in sickness, until death appears on the horizon. And we would all be poorer for that. A man who can leave his wife the day after she learns she has cancer, on the grounds that he has his own life to live, is to be deplored. The emotional inability or principled refusal to separate ourselves and our lives from the lives of ill or dying members of our families is *not* an unfortunate fact about the structure of our emotions. It is a desirable feature, not to be changed even if it could be; not to be changed even if the resulting intertwining of lives debars us from making exclusively self-regarding treatment decisions when we are ill.

Our present individualistic medical ethics is isolating and destructive. For by implicitly suggesting that patients make "their own" treatment decisions on a self-regarding basis and supporting those who do so, such an ethics encourages each of us to see our lives as simply our own. We may yet turn ourselves into beings who are ultimately alone.

FIDELITY OR FAIRNESS?

Fidelity to the interests of the patient has been a cornerstone of both traditional codes and contemporary theories of medical ethics. The two competing paradigms of medical ethics—the "benevolence" model and the "patient autonomy" model—are simply different ways of construing such fidelity. Both must be rejected or radically modified. The admission that treatment decisions often affect more than just the patient thus forces major changes on both the theoretical and the practical level. Obviously, I can only begin to explore the needed changes here.

Instead of starting with our usual assumption that physicians are to serve the interests of the patient, we must build our theories on a very different assumption: The medical and nonmedical interests of both the patient and other members of the patient's family are to be considered. It is only in the special case of patients without family that we can simply follow the patient's wishes or pursue the patient's interests. In fact, I would argue that we must build our theory of medical ethics on the presumption of equality: The interests of patients and family members are morally to be weighed equally; medical and nonmedical interests of the same magnitude deserve equal consideration in making treatment decisions. Like any other moral presumption, this one can, perhaps, be defeated in some cases. But the burden of proof will always be on those who would advocate special consideration for any family member's interests, including those of the ill.

Even where the presumption of equality is not defeated, life, health, and freedom from pain and handicapping conditions are extremely important goods for virtually everyone. They are thus very important considerations in all treatment decisions. In the majority of cases, the patient's interest in optimal health and longer life may well be strong enough to outweigh the conflicting interests of other members of the family. But even then, some departure from the treatment plan that would maximize the patient's interests may well be justified to harmonize best the interests of all concerned or to require significantly smaller sacrifices by other family members. That the patient's interests may often outweigh the conflicting interests of others in treatment decisions is no justification for failing to recognize that an attempt to balance or harmonize different, conflicting interests is often morally required. Nor does it justify overlooking the morally crucial cases in which the interests of other members of the family ought to override the interests of the patient. Changing our basic assumption about how treatment decisions are to be made means reconceptualizing the ethical roles of both physician and patient, since our understanding of both has been built on the presumption of patient primacy, rather than fairness to all concerned. Recognizing the moral relevance of the interests of family members thus reveals a dilemma for our understanding of what it is to be a physician: Should we retain a fiduciary ethic in which the physician is to serve the interests of her patient? Or should the physician attempt to weigh and balance all the interests of all concerned? I do not yet know just how to resolve this dilemma. All I can do here is try to envision the options.

If we retain the traditional ethic of fidelity to the interests of the patient, the physician should excuse herself from making treatment decisions that will affect the lives of the family on grounds of a moral conflict of interest, for she is a one-sided advocate. A lawyer for one of the parties cannot also serve as judge in the case. Thus, it would be unfair if a physician conceived as having a fiduciary relationship to her patient were to make treatment decisions that would adversely affect the lives of the patient's family. Indeed, a physician conceived as a patient advocate should not even *advise* patients or family members about which course of treatment should be chosen. As advocate, she can speak only to what course of treatment would be best for the patient, and must remain silent about what's best for the rest of the family or what should be done in light of everyone's interests.

Physicians might instead renounce their fiduciary relationship with their patients. On this view, physicians would no longer be agents of their patients and would not strive to be advocates for their patients' interests. Instead, the physician would aspire to be an impartial advisor who would stand knowledgeably but sympathetically outside all the many conflicting interests of those affected by the treatment options, and who would strive to discern the treatment that would best harmonize or balance the interests of all concerned.

Although this second option contradicts the Hippocratic oath and most other codes of medical ethics, it is not, perhaps, as foreign as it may at first seem. Traditionally, many family physicians—especially small-town physicians who knew patients and their families well—attempted to attend to both medical and nonmedical interests of all concerned. Many contemporary physicians still make decisions in this way. But we do not yet have an ethical theory that explains and justifies what they are doing.

Nevertheless, we may well question the physician's ability to act as an impartial ethical observer. Increasingly, physicians do not know their patients, much less their patients' families. Moreover, we may doubt physicians' abilities to weigh evenhandedly medical and nonmedical interests. Physicians are trained to be especially responsive to medical interests and we may well want them to remain that way. Physicians also tend to be deeply involved with the interests of their patients, and it may be impossible or undesirable to break this tie to enable physicians to be more impartial advisors. Finally, when someone retains the services of a physician, it seems reasonable that she be able to expect that physician to be *her* agent, pursuing *her* interests, not those of her family.

AUTONOMY AND ADVOCACY

We must also rethink our conception of the patient. On one hand, if we continue to stress patient autonomy, we must recognize that this implies that patients have moral responsibilities. If, on the other hand, we do not want to burden patients with weighty moral responsibilities, we must abandon the ethic of patient autonomy.

Recognizing that moral responsibilities come with patient autonomy will require basic changes in the accepted meanings of both "autonomy" and "advocacy." Because medical ethics has ignored patient responsibilities, we have come to interpret "autonomy" in a sense very different from Kant's original use of the term. It has come to mean simply the patient's freedom or right to choose the treatment he believes is best for himself. But as Kant knew well, there are many situations in which people can achieve autonomy and moral well-being only by sacrificing other important dimensions of their well-being, including health, happiness, even life itself. For autonomy is the *responsible* use of freedom and is therefore diminished whenever one ignores, evades, or slights one's responsibilities. Human dignity, Kant concluded, consists in our ability to refuse to compromise our autonomy to achieve the kinds of lives (or treatments) we want for ourselves.

If, then, I am morally empowered to make decisions about "my" medical treatment, I am also morally required to shoulder the responsibility of making very difficult moral decisions. The right course of action for me to take will not always be the one that promotes my own interests.

Some patients, motivated by a deep and abiding concern for the well-being of their families, will undoubtedly consider the interests of other family members. For these patients, the interests of their family are *part* of their interests. But not all patients will feel this way. And the interests of family members are not relevant *if* and *because* the patient wants to consider them; they are not relevant because they are *part* of the patient's interests. They are relevant *whether or not* the patient is inclined to consider them. Indeed, the *ethics* of patient decisions is most poignantly highlighted precisely when the patient is inclined to decide without considering the impact of his decision on the lives of the rest of his family.

Confronting patients with tough ethical choices may be part and parcel of treating them with respect as fully competent adults. We don't, after all, think it's right to stand silently by while other (healthy) adults ignore or shirk their moral responsibilities. If, however, we believe that most patients, gripped as they often are by the emotional crisis of serious illness, are not up to shouldering the responsibility of such decisions or should not be burdened with it, then I think we must simply abandon the ethic of patient autonomy. Patient autonomy would then be appropriate only when the various treatment options will affect only the patient's life.

The responsibilities of patients imply that there is often a conflict between patient autonomy and the patient's interests (even as those interests are defined by the patient). And we will have to rethink our understanding of patient advocacy in light of this conflict: Does the patient advocate try to promote the patient's (self-defined) *interests?* Or does she promote the patient's *autonomy* even at the expense of those interests? Responsible patient advocates can hardly encourage patients to shirk their moral responsibilities. But can we really expect health care providers to promote patient autonomy when that means encouraging their patients to sacrifice health, happiness, sometimes even life itself?

If we could give an affirmative answer to this last question, we would obviously thereby create a third option for reinterpreting the role of the physician: The physician could maintain her traditional role as patient advocate without being morally required to refrain from making treatment decisions whenever interests of the patient's family are also at stake *if* patient advocacy were understood as promoting patient autonomy *and* patient autonomy were understood as the responsible use of freedom, not simply the right to choose the treatment one wants.

Much more attention needs to be paid to all of these issues. However, it should be clear that absolutely central features of our theories of medical ethics—our understanding of physician and patient, and thus of patient advocacy as well as patient dignity, and patient autonomy—have presupposed that the interests of family members should be irrelevant or should always take a back seat to the interests of the patient. Basic conceptual shifts are required once we acknowledge that this assumption is not warranted.

Who Should Decide?

Such basic conceptual shifts will necessarily have ramifications that will be felt throughout the field of medical ethics, for a host of new and very different issues are raised by the inclusion of family interests. Discussions of privacy and confidentiality, of withholding/withdrawing treatment, and of surrogate decision making will all have to be reconsidered in light of the interests of the family. Many individual treatment decisions will also be affected, becoming much more complicated than they already are. Here, I will only offer a few remarks about treatment decisions, organized around the central issue of who should decide.

There are at least five answers to the question of who should make treatment decisions in cases where important interests of other family members are also at stake: the patient, the family, the physician, an ethics committee, or the courts. The physician's role in treatment decisions has already been discussed. Resorting to either the courts or to ethics committees for treatment decisions is too cumbersome and time-consuming for any but the most troubling cases. So I will focus here on the contrast between the patient and the family as appropriate decision makers. It is worth noting, though, that we need not arrive at one, uniform answer to cover all cases. On the contrary, each of the five options will undoubtedly have its place, depending on the particulars of the case at hand.

Should we still think of a patient as having the right to make decisions about "his" treatment? As we have seen, patient autonomy implies patient responsibilities. What, then, if the patient seems to be ignoring the impact of his treatment on his family? At the very least, responsible physicians must caution such patients against simply opting for treatments because they want them. Instead, physicians must speak of responsibilities and obligations. They must raise considerations of the quality of many lives, not just that of the patient. They must explain the distinction between making a decision and making it in a self-regarding manner. Thus, it will often be appropriate to make plain to patients the consequences of treatment decisions for their families and to urge them to consider these consequences in reaching a decision. And sometimes, no doubt, it will be appropriate for family members to present their cases to the patient in the hope that his decisions would be shaped by their appeals.

Nonetheless, we sometimes permit people to make bad or irresponsible decisions and *excuse* those decisions because of various pressures they were under when they made their choices. Serious illness can undoubtedly be an extenuating circumstance, and perhaps we should allow some patients to make some self-regarding decisions, especially if they insist on doing so and the negative impact of their decisions on others is not too great.

Alternatively, if we doubt that most patients have the ability to make treatment decisions that are really fair to all concerned, or if we are not prepared to accept a policy that would assign patients the responsibility of doing so, we may conclude that they should not be empowered to make treatment decisions in which the lives of their family members will be dramatically affected. Indeed, even if the patient were completely fair in making the decision, the autonomy of other family members would have been systematically undercut by the fact that the patient alone decided.

Thus, we need to consider the autonomy of all members of the family, not just the patient's autonomy. Considerations of fairness and, paradoxically, of autonomy therefore indicate that the *family* should make the treatment decision, with all competent family members whose lives will be affected participating. Many such family conferences undoubtedly already take place. On this view, however, family conferences would often be morally *required*. And these conferences would not be limited to cases involving incompetent patients; cases involving competent patients would also often require family conferences.

Obviously, it would be completely unworkable for a physician to convene a family conference every time a medical decision might have some ramifications on the lives of family members. However, such discussion need not always take place in the presence of the physician; we can recognize that formal family conferences become more important as the impact of treatment decisions on members of the patient's family grows larger. Family conferences may thus be morally *required* only when the lives of family members would be dramatically affected by treatment decisions.

Moreover, family discussion is often morally *desirable* even if not morally required. Desirable, sometimes, even for relatively minor treatment decisions: After the family has moved to a new town, should parents commit themselves to two-hour drives so that their teenage son can continue to be treated for his acne by the dermatologist he knows and whose results he trusts? Or should he seek treatment from a new dermatologist?

Some family conferences about treatment decisions would be characterized throughout by deep affection, mutual understanding, and abiding concern for the interests of others. Other conferences might begin in an atmosphere charged with antagonism, suspicion, and hostility but move toward greater understanding, reconciliation, and harmony within the family. Such conferences would be significant goods in themselves, as well as means to ethically better treatment decisions. They would leave all family members better able to go on with their lives.

Still, family conferences cannot be expected always to begin with or move toward affection, mutual understanding, and a concern for all. If we opt for joint treatment decisions when the lives of several are affected, we need to face the fact that family conferences will sometimes be bitter confrontations in which past hostilities, anger, and resentments will surface. Sometimes, too, the conflicts of interest between patient and family, and between one family member and another will be irresolvable, forcing families to invoke the harsh perspective of justice, divisive and antagonistic though that perspective may be. Those who favor family decisions when the whole family is affected will have to face the question of whether we really want to put the patient, already frightened and weakened by his illness, through the conflict and bitter confrontations that family conferences may sometimes precipitate.

We must also recognize that family members may be unable or unwilling to press or even state their own interests before a family member who is ill. Such refusal may be admirable, even heroic; it is sometimes evidence of willingness to go "above and beyond the call of duty," even at great personal cost. But not always. Refusal to press one's own interests can also be a sign of inappropriate guilt, of a crushing sense of responsibility for the well-being of others, of acceptance of an inferior or dominated role within the family, or of lack of a sense of self-worth. All of these may well be mobilized by an illness in the family. Moreover, we must not minimize the power of the medical setting to subordinate nonmedical to medical interests and to emphasize the well-being of the patient at the expense of the well-being of others. Thus, it will often be not just the patient, but also other family members who will need an advocate if a family conference is to reach the decision that best balances the autonomy and interests of all concerned.

The existing theory of patient autonomy and also of proxy decision making has been designed partly as a buttress against pressures from family members for both overtreatment and undertreatment of patients. The considerations I have been advancing will enable us to understand that sometimes what we've seen as undertreatment or overtreatment may not really be such. Both concepts will have to be redefined. Still, I do not wish to deny or minimize the problem of family members who demand inappropriate treatment. Treatment decisions are extremely difficult when important interests of the other members of the family are also at stake. The temptation of family members simply to demand the treatment that best suits *their* interests is often very real.

I do not believe, however, that the best safeguard against pressures from family members for inappropriate treatment is to issue morally inappropriate instructions to them in the hope that these instructions will prevent abuses. Asking a family member to pretend that her interests are somehow irrelevant often backfires. Rather, I think the best safeguard would be candidly to admit the moral relevance of the interests of other members of the family and then to support the family through the excruciating process of trying to reach a decision that is fair to all concerned.

Acknowledging the interests of family members in medical treatment decisions thus forces basic changes at the level of ethical theory and in the moral practice of medicine. The sheer complexity of the issues raised might seem a sufficient reason to ignore family interests in favor of the much simpler ethic of absolute fidelity to the patient. But that would be the ostrich approach to the complexities of medical ethics. We must not abandon our patients' families to lives truncated by an oversimplified ethic, for that would be an unconscionable toll to exact to make our tasks as ethicists and moral physicians easier.

Reconstructing medical ethics in light of family interests would not be all pain and no gain for ethicists and physicians. Acknowledging family members' interests would bring benefits as well as burdens to medical practitioners, for the practice of medicine has rarely been as individualistic as codes and theories of medical ethics have advocated. Indeed, much of what now goes on in intensive care nurseries, pediatricians' offices, intensive care units, and long-term care institutions makes ethical sense *only* on the assumption that the interests of other members of the family are also to be considered.

Contemporary ethical theory and traditional codes of medical ethics can neither help nor support physicians, patients, and family members struggling to balance the patient's interests and the interests of others in the family. Our present ethical theory can only condemn as unethical any attempt to weigh in the interests of other family members. If we would acknowledge the moral relevance of the interests of the family we could perhaps develop an ethical theory that would guide and support physicians, patients, and families in the throes of agonizing moral decisions.

ACKNOWLEDGMENTS

I wish to thank Mary Read English, Michael Lavin, Gary Smith, Joanne Lynn, and Larry Churchill for valuable suggestions.

The Problem of Proxies with Interests of Their Own

Toward a Better Theory of Proxy Decisions

A 78-year-old married woman with progressive Alzheimer's disease was admitted to a local hospital with pneumonia and other medical problems. She was able to recognize no one, and she had been incontinent for about a year. Despite aggressive treatment, the pneumonia failed to resolve, and it seemed increasingly likely that this admission was to be for terminal care. The patient's husband (who had been taking care of her in their home) began requesting that the doctors be less aggressive in their treatment and, as the days wore on, he became more and more insistent that they scale back their aggressive care. The physicians were reluctant to do so, due to the small but real chance that the patient could survive to discharge. The husband was the patient's only remaining family, so he was the logical proxy decision maker. Multiple conferences ensued; finally a conference with a social worker revealed that the husband had recently proposed marriage to the couple's housekeeper, and she had accepted.

THE CURRENT THEORY OF PROXY DECISIONS

Patient autonomy is the cornerstone of our medical ethics. Given this commitment to autonomy, proxy decisions will always strike us as problematic: It is always more difficult to ensure that the wishes of the patient are embodied in treatment decisions when someone else must speak for the patient. Proxy decisions are especially disturbing when we fear that the proxy's judgment is tainted by his own interests, so that the proxy is covertly requesting the treatment *he* wants the patient to have, rather than the treatment the *patient* would have wanted. This problem of interested proxies is exacerbated by the fact that we seek out proxies who often turn out to have strong interests in the treatment of the patient. We do this for two reasons: (1) Those who care deeply for the patient are more likely than others to want what is best for the patient. (2) Those who are close to the patient are generally most knowledgeable about what the patient would have wanted. This familiarity allows us to apply the *substituted-judgment* standard of proxy decision making. Given a commitment to autonomy, substituted judgment is an ethically better basis for proxy decision making than the *reasonable-person* or *best-interest* standard.

The apparent alternative would be proxy decisions made by outsiders—physicians, court-appointed guardians, or ethics committees. We must learn to recognize that such outsiders also have interests of their own, and that their proxy decisions may also be influenced by these interests. The more common worry about outsiders is that they rarely know the patient as well as members of the patient's family do, and outsiders' concern about the individual patient does not run nearly as deep. Proxies who are members of the patient's family have a difficult time ignoring their own interests in treatment decisions, precisely because they—unlike outsiders—are so intimately involved with the patient and have so much at stake.

Thus, it seems that our theory of proxy decisions has boxed us into a "Catch 22" situation. "Knowledgeable" about patient wishes usually means "close," but close almost always means having interests of one's own in the case. "Disinterested" usually means "distant," and distance usually brings with it less real concern, as well as lack of the intimate knowledge required to render a reliable substituted judgment.

I will argue that the reservations we have about interested family members and their proxy decisions are partly of our own making. The accepted theory of proxy decisions is deeply flawed and must be recast. Our medical practice is, I believe, often better than the conventional theories of proxy decision making. Nonetheless, some of our deepest worries about proxy decision makers grow out of the morally inappropriate instructions we give them.

If the current theory about proxy decisions for incompetent patients is mistaken, the accepted view of decisions by *competent* patients will have to be modified as well. However, I will be able to discuss decisions by competent patients only very briefly at the end of the article.

CASE ANALYSIS: THE HUSBAND AND HIS PROXY DECISION

The husband in this case seemed a perfect scoundrel. The physicians involved in the case all believed that he should be disqualified as a proxy decision maker, due to his obvious conflict of interest and his patent inability to ignore his own interests in making decisions about his wife's care. There was no reason to believe that the patient would have wanted to limit her treatment, so the conclusion seemed inescapable that the husband was not faithfully discharging his role as proxy decider.

Both traditional codes and contemporary theories of medical ethics hold that physicians are obligated to deliver treatment that reflects the wishes or the best interest of the patient, and that the incompetence of the patient does nothing to alter this obligation.[1] There is similar unanimity about the responsibilities of a proxy decision maker: The proxy decision maker is to make the treatment decisions that most faithfully reflect the patient's wishes or, if those wishes cannot be known, the best interest of the patient.[2] If the proxy does not do so, commentators almost uniformly recommend that physicians reject the proxy's requests and have recourse to an ethics committee or to the courts.

Despite this impressive consensus of both traditional codes and contemporary theories of medical ethics, I was intrigued by this case and pressed the attending physician for more details. "Why is the husband in such a hurry? Perhaps he hopes that his wife will die, but she is dying anyway. Is he afraid that she might not die?" "No," the attending responded, "his worries are primarily financial. He is afraid that he'll lose his house and all his savings to medical bills before she dies. Since the housekeeper has no assets, they will then be left poverty-stricken."

To some, this seems even worse: The husband has not only allowed his own interests to override considerations of what is best for his wife, but he has let his own crass financial considerations predominate. If his decision is not altogether self-centered, it is only because he is concerned about his fiancee's future as well as his own. But married men are not supposed to have fiancees.

I do not necessarily want to argue that the husband made the correct decision. And I do not know enough about him to be able to judge his character. But I do think his decision should not be rejected out-of-hand, as patently inappropriate. First, I do not believe that we can just assume that the presence of another woman means that he was insensitive to his wife's interests. I certainly know couples who have gotten divorced without losing the ability to care genuinely about each other and each other's interests. Second, while divorcing a long-standing wife simply because she is now demented is difficult—"How can I abandon her at a time when she is so vulnerable?"—remaining married to an increasingly unreachable, foreign woman with Alzheimer's is difficult, too. His wife's dementia undoubtedly meant increasing isolation for him, as well as for her. And given that reality, his search for companionship does not seem unreasonable or morally objectionable. Third, the husband also had been the patient's primary caregiver for years without any prospect of relief or improvement. He probably longed for a chance to spend his few remaining years free of the burdens of such care. And, finally, supposing the husband to be an adherent of traditional values, he would be able to bring himself neither to simply "live with" the housekeeper, nor to consider himself no longer married while his wife was still alive, nor to accept medical care with no intention of trying to pay for it. Perhaps more "liberal" attitudes toward marriage and the payment of debts would have served his wife better. But we cannot be sure about that.

I have no doubt that the husband's proxy decisions were influenced by his own interests. Given the reasonableness and magnitude of the interests he had at stake, it is hard to see how he could ignore them. "How can *we* ignore his interests?" I wondered. "And how can we reasonably ask him to ignore them?" I do not think we can.

The attending physician and I got no further on this case than my suggestion that the husband's concern about his financial future was an appropriate consideration in deciding on a course of treatment for the patient. The physician was shocked that I thought this kind of consideration was relevant.

However, in today's society we limit treatment all the time in an effort to save money for the government or for a health maintenance organization. We develop theories of rationing and "costworthy" medicine to justify such decisions.[3] We regularly deinstitutionalize people, partly to limit the cost of the care that we, as a society, must provide. We limit the number of nursing home beds available for this man's wife and other Alzheimer's victims for the same reason. We thus force the burden of long-term care onto the families of the ill. And then we tell them that they must not consider their own burdens in making treatment decisions. I cannot make ethical sense of this.

We consider *our* pocketbooks, so how can we in good conscience tell proxies that they must ignore the impact of aggressive treatment on their personal financial futures? Financial considerations for a 75-year-old with limited means are never trivial. We must recognize that for him, nothing less is at stake than the quality of the rest of his life, including, quite likely, the quality of his own future health care.

If we find it morally repugnant that proxies decide to limit treatment due to the burdens of long-term care on the family, then it is incumbent upon us to devise an alternative to our present system under which families deliver 75 percent of the long-term care. And until we have such an alternative in place, we dare not direct the husband to ignore the impact of treatment decisions on his own life. For *we* do not ignore the impact of such decisions on our lives. Moreover, the burdens of his wife's treatment to him may well outweigh any benefits we might be able to provide for her.

THE MORAL RELEVANCE OF FAMILY MEMBERS' INTERESTS

There are, of course, many cases like this, in which optimal care for a patient will result in diminished quality of life for those close to the patient. This care can be a crushing financial burden, depriving other family members of many different goods and opportunities. But the burdens are by no means only financial: Caring for an aging parent with decreasing mental capabilities or a severely retarded child with multiple medical problems can easily become the social and emotional center of a family's existence, draining away time and energy from all other facets of life. What are we to say about such cases?

I submit that we must acknowledge that many treatment decisions inevitably and dramatically affect the quality of more lives than one. This is true for a variety of very different reasons: (1) People get emotionally involved with others, and whatever affects the people we love affects us, too. (2) People live together, and important changes in one member of a living unit will usually have ramifications for all the others, as well. (3) The family is a financial unit in our culture, and treatment decisions often carry important financial implications that can radically limit the life plans of the rest of the family. (4)

Marriage and the family are also legal relationships, and one's legal status hinges on the life or death of other members of the family. (5) Treatment decisions have an important impact on the lives of others, because we are loyal to one another.

Most of us do not believe that family and friendships are to be dissolved whenever their continued existence threatens one's quality of life. I know of a man who left his wife the day after she learned that she had cancer, because living with a cancer-stricken woman was no part of his vision of the good life. But most of us are unable or unwilling to disentangle ourselves and our lives from others when continuing involvement threatens the quality of our own lives.

This loyalty is undoubtedly a good thing. Without it, we would have alliances for better but not for worse, in health but not in sickness, until death appears on the horizon. It is a good thing even though it sometimes brings about one of the really poignant ironies of human existence: Sometimes it is precisely this loyalty that gives rise to insoluble and very basic conflicts of interest, as measures to promote the quality of one life undermine the quality of others. If the husband in the case we have been considering had simply divorced his wife when she was diagnosed as having Alzheimer's, she would have died utterly alone. As such, only her own interests would have been relevant to her treatment. Her husband's loyalty—impure though it may have been—has undoubtedly made her life with Alzheimer's much better for her. But it also makes her treatment not simply her own.

Now, if medical treatment decisions will often dramatically affect the lives of more than one, I submit that we cannot morally disregard the impact of those decisions on all lives except the patient's. Nor can we justify making the interests of the patient predominant by claiming that medical interests should always take precedence over other interests. Life and health are important goods in the lives of almost everyone. Consequently, health-related considerations are often important enough to override the interests of family members in treatment decisions. But not always. Even life or death is not always the most important consideration. Thus, although persons become "patients" in medical settings, and medical settings are organized around issues of life and health, we must still bear in mind that these are not always the most important considerations. We must beware of the power of the medical context to subordinate all other interests to medical interests. Sometimes nonmedical interests of nonpatients morally ought to take precedence over medical interests of patients.

Because medical treatment decisions often deeply affect more lives than one, proxy decision makers must consider the ramifications of treatment decisions on all those who will be importantly affected, including themselves. Everyone with important interests at stake has a morally legitimate claim to consideration; no one's interests can be ignored or left out of consideration. And this means nothing less than that the morally best treatment in many cases will not be the treatment that is best for the patient.

An exclusively patient-centered ethics must be abandoned. It must be abandoned, not only—as is now often acknowledged—because of scarce medical resources and society's limited ability to meet virtually unlimited demands for medical treatment. It must be abandoned, as well, because it is patently unfair to the families of patients. And if this is correct, the current theory of proxy decisions must be rejected in favor of an ethics that attempts to harmonize and balance the interests of friends and family whose lives will be deeply affected by the patient's treatment.[4]

REEXAMINING THE DOCTRINE OF SUBSTITUTED JUDGMENT

There is a second, related point. Arguably, there is a presumption that substituted judgment is a morally appropriate standard for a proxy decision maker. But this can be no more than a *presumption*, and it can be overridden whenever various treatment options will affect the lives of the patient's family. In fact, substituted judgment is the appropriate standard for proxy decision making in only two special (though not uncommon) situations: (1) when the treatment decision will affect only the patient, or (2) when the patient's judgment would have duly reflected the interests of others whose lives will be affected. In other situations, proxy deciders should make decisions that may be *at odds with* the known wishes of a formerly competent patient.

Consider again the case with which this paper began. I did not know the patient, and I have no idea what kind of a person she used to be. Let us, then, consider two rather extreme hypotheses about her character. On one hand, suppose that the patient had been a very selfish, domineering woman who, throughout their marriage, had always been willing to subordinate her husband's interests to her own. If so, we can reliably infer that she would now have ignored her husband's interests again, perhaps even ridden roughshod over them, if she could have gotten something she wanted by doing so. Therefore, we can conclude that she would have demanded all the medical treatment available, regardless of costs to him. We can even imagine that she would have relished her continuing power over him and her ability to continue to extract sacrifices from him. Obviously, her husband would know these facts about her. The substituted-judgment standard of proxy decisions would have us conclude that if that is the kind of woman she was, this would *increase* her husband's obligation to make additional sacrifices of his interests to hers.

Suppose, on the other hand, that this woman had always been a generous, considerate, unselfish woman who was deeply sensitive to the interests of her husband and always ready to put his needs before her own. If that is the kind of woman she was, the theory of substituted judgment allows—strictly speaking, even *obligates*—her husband to sacrifice her interests once again by now demanding minimal care for her. After all, he knows that is what she would have done, had she been competent to make the decision. Even if he wanted to give her the very best treatment as an expression of love or gratitude for her concern for him throughout their lives, substituted judgment would require that he ignore those desires. Continued treatment is what *he* wants for her, not what she would have chosen for herself.

But surely that is exactly wrong. The theory of substituted judgment has it backwards. Loving, giving, generous people deserve to be generously cared for when they can no longer make decisions for themselves, even if they would not have been generous with themselves. And what do selfish, domineering, tyrannical people deserve? The answer to that question depends on one's ethical theory. Perhaps neglect, maybe even retribution, are justified or at least excusable. Perhaps tyrannical behavior releases the family from any special obligation to care for the now incompetent tyrant. But unless one believes that good people should not be rewarded for their virtues, one will agree that caring, giving individuals deserve better care than domineering, self-centered individuals.

Where did we go wrong? What led us to widespread acceptance of the theory of substituted judgment? The major mistake is the one we have been considering—the mistake of believing that medical treatment affects only the life of the patient, or that its impact on other lives should be ignored. If the patient's interests are the only ones that ought to shape treatment decisions, those interests are best defined by the patient's point of view. Proxy deciders are, then, obligated to replicate that point of view insofar as possible. But most decisions we make affect the lives of others. That, of course, is the main reason why we have ethics. And the present incompetence of a patient should not obligate others to perpetuate the patient's former selfish ways.

It would, of course, be possible to modify and defend the doctrine of substituted judgment by reinterpreting the concept of autonomy.[5] Patient autonomy is, after all, the main reason we embrace substituted judgment, and we usually define patient autonomy as "what the patient would have wanted." But if we were to work instead with a truly Kantian notion of autonomy, we would arrive at a very different theory of substituted judgment. For Kant would insist that a domineering, selfish person would acknowledge that she deserves less generous care when she becomes incompetent than a more caring, giving person deserves. While she might not actually elect less generous care if she were able to choose for herself, the moral judge within her would recognize that she deserves less care from others due to the way she has treated them.

On Kant's view, then, the treatment she would choose for herself is not the appropriate standard of autonomy. Rather, her judgment about what is fair or what she now deserves would be the true meaning of autonomy. Kant would insist that the selfish, domineering ways of an individual are all heteronomous (subject to external influences), despite the fact that the person consistently chose them. He would further insist that a request for medical care that requires inordinate sacrifices from one's family is also heteronomous, even if the patient would have wanted that. This interpretation of autonomy and substituted judgment is clearly very different from the standard interpretation in medical ethics.

Barring a radical rethinking of the very concepts of autonomy and substituted judgment, the doctrine of substituted judgment must be rejected. At the very least, our standard view of substituted judgment must be replaced with a theory in which the interests of the incompetent are constrained by what is morally appropriate, *whether or not* the patient would have so constrained herself. Often, the patient would have been sensitive to the interests of the rest of the family. But not always. In any case, the interests of other members of the family are not relevant to proxy decisions *because* the patient would have considered them as part of her own interests; they are relevant *whether or not* the patient would have considered them.[6] It is simply not the patient's regard for the interests of her family that gives those interests moral standing. No patient, competent or incompetent, deserves more than a fair, equitable consideration of the interests of all concerned. Fairness to all includes, I would add, fairness to the patient herself, in light of the life she has lived and especially the way she has treated the members of her family.

The theory of proxy decision making must be rebuilt. While proxy deciders must guard against *undue* consideration of their own interests, undue consideration of the *patient's* interests is likewise to be avoided. Proxy deciders have been given the wrong instructions. Instead of telling them that they must attempt to put themselves into the shoes of the incompetent patient and decide as she would have decided, we must tell them that the incompetent patient's wishes are the best way to define *her* interests, but what she would have wanted for herself must be balanced against considerations of fairness to all members of the family.

Toward a New Theory of Proxy Decisions

Fundamental changes in the theory of proxy decisions will need to be created and defended. And a view such as mine faces a host of important questions. I cannot develop an alternative theory in this article. Indeed, I cannot even fully answer the most pressing questions about an alternative. Here, I can only provide suggestions about the way I would try to approach four of the most immediate questions about the theory of proxy decisions I would advocate.

First, if proxy deciders must avoid *undue* consideration of either their own interests or the interests of the patient, how is "undue consideration" to be defined? A full answer to this question would require an account of the family and of the ethics of the family. We can begin, however, by noting that, *prima facie,* equal interests deserve equal consideration. But what defines equal interest? Norman Daniels has developed the concept of a "normal opportunity range" for the purpose of allocating resources to different individuals and different age groups.[7] Perhaps this concept could be extended to problems of fairness *within* families by asking how different treatment options will affect the opportunity range of the various members of the family. If so, undue consideration could be partially defined as a bias in favor of an interest that affects someone's opportunity range in a smaller way over an interest that affects another's opportunity range in a greater way.

But even if this suggestion about the opportunity range could be worked out, it would represent only one dimension of an adequate account of undue consideration. Another dimension would be fairness to competent and formerly competent members of the family in light of the way they have lived and treated each other. Thus, as I have argued earlier, those who have been caring and generous to members of their families deserve more from them than those who have been selfish or inconsiderate.

Second, *whose* interests are to be considered? For example, what about the interests of family members who do not care for the patient or who have long been hostile to the patient? Lack of concern for the patient and even hostility toward the patient do not, on my view, exclude family members from consideration. Such family members still may have important interests at stake; moreover, we must not assume that the neglect or hostility is not merited. Neglect or hostility toward the patient would, however, diminish what fair consideration of their interests would amount to.

What of the interests of close friends or companions who are not members of the family? "Family," as I intend this concept, is not restricted to blood or marital relationships. Close friends, companions, unmarried lovers—all of these relationships may entitle persons to consideration in treatment decisions. Those who are distant—neither emotionally involved with the patient nor related by blood or marriage—will almost never have strong enough interests in the treatment of a patient to warrant consideration. (Health care professionals may have strong interests, but they have special professional obligations to ignore their own interests and are usually well compensated for doing so.) I see no principled way to exclude consideration of anyone whose interests will be importantly affected by a treatment decision.

Third, wouldn't any theory like the one I propose result in unfair treatment of incompetent patients? After all, we do not require that competent patients consider the interests of their families when making treatment decisions. And if competent patients can ignore their families, doesn't fairness require that we permit incompetent patients to do so, as well? I have argued elsewhere that if we want to insist on patient autonomy, we must insist that patients have *responsibilities* and *obligations,* as well.[8] In many cases, it is irresponsible and wrong for competent patients to make self-centered or exclusively self-regarding treatment decisions. It is often wrong for a competent patient to consider only which treatment she wants for herself. We must, then, try to figure out what to do when patients abuse their autonomy—when they disregard the impact of their treatment decisions on the lives of others. Sometimes, no doubt, we should seek to find ways to prevent patients from abusing their autonomy at too great a cost to their families.

Still, competent patients are almost always permitted to ignore the interests of their family members, even when this is wrong. We do not force them to consider the impact of their decisions on others, nor do we disallow their decisions if they fail to do so. How, then, can it be fair to incompetent patients to develop a theory of proxy decisions that will, in effect, hold them to a more stringent moral standard by requiring them to accept treatment decisions made in light of their families' interests? The answer to this question is, I think, that there are many actions that we are at liberty to take, but only so long as we do not need an agent to help us accomplish them. If we can file our own taxes, we may be able to cheat in ways that a responsible tax advisor will refuse to do. We may get away with shoddy deals that an ethical lawyer would not be a party to. Thus, the greater freedom of competent patients is only a special case of the generally greater freedom of action when no assistance of an agent is required.

And fourth, what about the legal difficulties of an alternative view of proxy decision making? They are considerable: It is presently *illegal* to make proxy decisions in the way I think is morally appropriate. The courts that have become involved in proxy decisions have almost all opted for exclusively patient-centered standards. I do not have the expertise needed to address the legal issues my view raises. My purpose here can only be to challenge the faulty moral foundations that undergird present legal practice.

However, it is possible that family law could provide a model for a revised legal standard of proxy decision making. Family law recognizes the legitimacy of proxy decisions—for children, for example—that are not always in the best interest of the person represented by the proxy. It has to, if only because there are many cases in which the interests of one child will conflict with those of others. Nor does family law require parents to ignore their own interests in deciding for a child; instead, it defines standards of minimum acceptable care, with the hope that most families will do better than these minimum standards. Perhaps we should similarly separate the legal from the moral standard for proxy decisions. If no abuse or neglect is involved, the legal standard is met, though that may be less than morality requires of a proxy decision maker.

CONCLUSION

All these issues—undue consideration, eligible interests, fairness between competent and incompetent patients, and the law of proxy decisions—may seem very complex. However, I do not believe they are unnecessarily complicated. Many important decisions within families are very complicated. In medical ethics, we have simplified our task by working with an artificially oversimplified vision of the interests and decisions of families in medical treatment. So, if my critique of the present theory of proxy decisions is correct, we all—medical ethicists, reflective health care practitioners, legal theorists, lawyers—have a lot of hard work to do. The change I propose is basic, so the revisions required will be substantial.

I close now with a word of caution and a word of encouragement. The word of caution: We must recognize that even the necessary revisions in our moral and legal theories of proxy decisions would not resolve all the problems of proxy decisions. Proxy deciders with interests that conflict with those of the patient do face serious moral difficulties and very real temptations to give undue weight to their own interests. Although the concepts of both "overtreatment" and "undertreatment" will have to be redefined in light of the considerations I have been advancing, pressure from proxies for inappropriate treatment will remain. I do not wish to minimize these difficulties in any way.

But we should not give proxies the morally erroneous belief that their own interests are irrelevant, censuring them for allowing their interests to "creep in" to their decisions. Instead, we must deal forthrightly with the very real difficulties arising from interested proxy decisions, by making these interests conscious, explicit, and legitimate. Then we must provide guidance and support for those caught in the moral crucible of proxy decisions. Not only would this approach be more ethically sound, but it would, I believe, decrease the number of inappropriate proxy decisions.

Finally, an encouraging word. The Alzheimer's case that I have cited notwithstanding, the practice of medicine is often better than our ethical theories have been. It has generally not been so insensitive to the interests of family members as our theories would ask that it be. Indeed, much of what now goes on in intensive care nurseries, pediatricians' offices, intensive care units, and long-term care facilities makes ethical sense *only* on the assumption that fairness to the interests of the other members of the family is morally required. To mention only the most obvious kind of case, I have never seen a discussion about institutional versus home care for an incompetent patient that did not attempt to address the interests of those who would have to care for the patient, as well as the interests of the patient.

Current ethical theory and traditional codes of medical ethics can neither help nor support health care professionals and proxies struggling to balance the patient's interests with those of the proxy and other family members. Indeed, our present ethical theory can only condemn as unethical any attempt to weigh in the interests of the family. Thus, our ethical theory forces us to misdescribe decisions about institutionalization in terms of what is physically or psychologically possible for the family, rather than in terms of what is or is not too much to ask of them. If we were to acknowledge the moral relevance and legitimacy of the family's interests, we would be able to understand why many treatment decisions now being made make sense and are not unethical. And then we would be in a position to develop an ethical theory that would guide health care providers and proxies in the throes of excruciating moral decisions.

ACKNOWLEDGMENTS

I wish to thank Eric H. Loewy and especially Mary R. English for many helpful comments on this paper.

NOTES

1. L. Edelstein, "The Hippocratic Oath: Text, Translation and Interpretation," *Bulletin of the History of Medicine*, supp. 1. Baltimore: Johns Hopkins University Press, 1943, 3; World Medical Association, "Declaration of Geneva." *World Medical Journal* 3, supp. (1956): 10–12; World Medical Association, "International Code of Medical Ethics," *World Medical Association Bulletin* I (1949): 109–11; T. L. Beauchamp, and J. F. Childress, Principles of Biomedical Ethics, 3rd ed. New York: Oxford University Press, 1989; A. E. Buchanan, and D. W. Brock, *Deciding for Others: The Ethics of Surrogate Decision Making*, New York: Cambridge UP, 1989; J. F. Childress. *Who Should Decide? Paternalism in Health Care*, (New York: Oxford, University Press, 1982; Hastings Center, *Guidelines on the Termination of Life-Sustaining Treatment and the Care of the Dying*, Bloomington, IN: Indiana University Press, 1987; E. D. Pellegrino, and D.

C. Thomasma. *For the Patient's Good*. New York: Oxford UP, 1988; President's Commission for the Study of Ethical Problems in Medicine and Biomedical and Behavioral Research. *Making Health Care Decisions: The Ethical and Legal Implications of Informed Consent in the Patient-Physician Relationship*, vol. 1. Washington, DC: US Government Printing Office, 1982; Veatch, R. M. A Theory of Medical Ethics. New York: Basic Books, 1981.

2. Beauchamp and Childress, *Principles of Biomedical Ethics*; Buchanan and Brock, *Deciding for Others*; Hastings Center, *Guidelines*; Pellegrino and Thomasma, *For the Patient's Good*; President's Commission, *Making Health Care Decisions*; R. M. Veatch. *Death, Dying and the Biological Revolution: Our Last Quest for Responsibility*, New Haven, CT: Yale UP, 1989.

3. See, for example, D. Callahan. *Setting Limits: Medical Goals in an Aging Society*. (New York: Simon and Schuster, 1987); N. Daniels. *Just Health Care* (New York: Cambridge UP, 1985); R. W. Evans. "Health Care Technology and the Inevitability of Resource Allocation and Rationing Decisions (pt. 2)." *Journal of the American Medical Association* 249 (1983): 2208–19; E. H. Morreim. "Fiscal Scarcity and the Inevitability of Bedside Budget Balancing." *Archives of Internal Medicine* 149 (1989): 1012–15; R. M. Veatch. "Justice and the Economics of Terminal Illness." *Hastings Center Report* 18 (August-September 1988): 34–40; L. C. Thurow. "Learning to Say 'No.' "*New England Journal of Medicine* 311 (1984): 1569–72.

4. There are a few scattered references that acknowledge that the interests of the patient's family may be considered. At one point, the President's Commission states that "the impact of a decision on an incapacitated patient's loved ones may be taken into account," (President's Commission for the Study of Ethical Problems in Medicine and Biomedical and Behavioral Research, *Deciding to Forego Life-Sustaining Treatment: Ethical, Medical and Legal Issues in Treatment Decisions*. Washington, DC: US Government Printing Office, 1983, 135–36). The Hastings Center Guidelines counsels consideration of the benefits and burdens to "the patient's family and concerned friends," but only in the special case of patients with irreversible loss of consciousness (p. 29). Buchanan and Brock devote one page of their impressive work, Deciding for Others, to the "limits on the burdens it is reasonable to expect family members to bear" (p. 208). But these are only isolated passages in large, systematic works and they do not inform the overall theory developed in these works. The discussion of neonatal care is the only place I know where the interests of members of the patient's family have received systematic attention. A good example is C. Strong. "The Neonatologist's Duty to Patients and Parents." *Hastings Center Report* 14 (August 1984): 10–16. The fact that many ethicists seem willing to consider family interests in the case of newborns but not in the case of older patients suggests that we may not really consider newborns to be full-fledged persons.

5. I owe this point to an anonymous referee.

6. Thus, I am in substantial disagreement with even the one paragraph from the President's Commission's Deciding to Forego Life-Sustaining Treatment that goes farthest toward something like the position I embrace. For the President's Commission would allow proxies to consider the interests of family members only if there is substantial evidence that the patient would have considered their interests. But on my view, this is not the reason that the interests of the members of the patient's family are relevant. If the patient was a selfish, inconsiderate person, this does not mean that the interests of her family somehow become morally illegitimate or irrelevant.

7. N. Daniels. *Just Health Care*. Cambridge England: Cambridge UP, 1985.

8. J. Hardwig. "What About the Family? The Role of Family Interests in Medical Treatment Decisions." *Hastings Center Report* 20 (March–April 1990): 5–10.

SUPPORT and the Invisible Family

"I just *have* to believe that my mother simply isn't aware of what she's doing to me and my life." The tone of weariness and near desperation in my friend Jane's voice made it clear that if she did not believe this, she would be filled with anger and resentment at her dying mother. Despite terminal heart disease, her mother, Helen, an 83-year-old former nurse, keeps opting for life-prolonging treatment. For the past 18 months, the hospital has pulled Helen through crisis after crisis, each time discharging her back home, lucid and grateful, and only slightly more dependent than she was before.

For millennia, medical ethics has focused on the doctor–patient relationship. Thus, the SUPPORT trial to improve clinical decision making for seriously ill patients can be viewed as a report about the failure of this dyadic relationship. That is the way I expect most people to read it. And there clearly *is* a failure of this dyad: physicians who are so unconcerned about patient preferences that they don't even bother to look at them when they're placed in the chart, and patients who do not take advantage of opportunities to discuss their treatment preferences with their physicians.

Helen's case, though, is different. Intelligent, articulate, and assertive, Helen has made her preferences for treatment very clear to her physicians and her wishes are being followed. The dyad seems to be working fine here.

If we look only at Helen, the story seems to be an unqualified success. A very difficult case (this woman might not have pulled through this episode) managed well. Discharged back home, still in a lucid state. End of the case, a job well done Congratulations all around for one of those spectacular successes of modern medicine.

But we need to understand Jane's weariness, frustration, anger, and resentment. These are not feelings generated by a simple success story with a happy ending. We must learn to tell the story from Jane's point of view and not to end the story when Helen is discharged. Jane's story is usually not heard. Helen has many advocates—doctors, nurses, ethics committees, most bioethicists, and our entire legal system. Jane will usually have none.

If Helen's case is viewed simply as Helen's case, Jane becomes invisible. The impact of the treatment on *her* life is not considered, her interests do not even enter the equation. At best, she is marginalized: Her interests are considered, but Helen's interests always trump Jane's. Often, she is treated as a means ("family support system") for helping her mother achieve her goal of continuing to live in her invalid state. Helen does have a strong family support system and that system is Jane. The home to which Helen is discharged is, in fact, Jane's home.

I cannot do justice to Jane's story here. But I will at least mention some of the things her mother's fight against death have meant for her. She has been driven to the edge of physical, emotional, and economic collapse. Her savings have been exhausted. The prospects for her own old age have been devastated–a 55 year-old with a modest income has too little time left in her employable life to rebuild a nest egg for retirement. Jane clings to a full-time job and another part-time job, desperately needing the money. She also knows that if she quits or is fired, she will have to relocate or change careers, neither a simple task for a single woman of her age. Fortunately, she can do much of her work at home, sandwiched between periods of caring for her mother. Jane has no social life now and no time to herself except during the periods when her mother is rehospitalized. That's also when she can get some rest. Jane's employers have begun to worry that Jane is not doing a very good job these days.

Viewed in terms of its impact on Jane's life, her mother's treatment is not a miracle of modern medicine, a triumph, or even a clear success. It is more like a disaster. Jane's story is not unusual—there are literally millions of people in similar circumstances. To their credit, the authors of the SUPPORT studies have not confined themselves to a dyadic or triadic ethics. In fact, they have documented at least the most measurable impacts of treatment decisions on families in a recent article in *JAMA*.[1] That part of the SUPPORT study deserves to be read in conjunction with this one.

Read by itself, this part of the SUPPORT study invites the wrong conclusions. The SUPPORT intervention asked physicians to take into consideration patient preferences and prognoses. The physicians failed to do so. Thus, this study strongly suggests that inappropriate treatment decisions are being made at the end of life and that they are being made by the wrong decision makers. I believe both are true. But if we think only in terms of the usual dyad or triad of bioethics, we may conclude that patient preferences and prognoses are the salient variables in defining appropriate treatment at the end of life. If this conclusion is drawn, families become invisible or are treated as means to the well-being of terminally ill patients.

How can we give patients' families their due? We can begin by at least acknowledging our responsibility for their plights. Those with a serious illness in their families are not simply people stuck in a bad situation. They are not just victims of unfortunate circumstances, bad luck, or cruel fate. Although an illness in the family may well be simply unfortunate, the treatment of that illness is something we decide. So, families are also the victims of our treatment decisions, our health care system, our bioethics. *We* have seriously compromised the lives of patients' families, often in ways they can never recover from. We must acknowledge as much.

We must also recognize that families are not simply or even primarily "patient support systems." They must not be thought of or treated that way by doctors, hospitals, health care planners, or bioethicists. To do so is immoral, as Kant made plain. It involves treating the rest of the patient's family as a mere means to the preferences of the patient. Others are implicitly treated as mere means whenever only one person's interests and goals are allowed to shape decisions that alter the lives of many people.

Everyone is an end in herself. The implications for the life plans of all family members must be weighed in responsible treatment decisions.

When this is done, the very definition of "appropriate treatment at the end of life" will be altered. If families are not marginalized, patients who survive to discharge back home in a lucid state cannot be viewed as unambiguous success stories. A treatment may be inappropriate even if the patient was treated according to her preferences and the cost was modest.

How modest is the cost, really? Cost to whom? Consider just the monetary costs. We are currently engaged in a badly needed effort to control health care costs. But if we think simply in terms of the triad, measures designed to save money will often simply shift much of the cost to the families of patients. Where they are, once again, largely invisible to us. *We* don't have to pay these costs, so we congratulate ourselves for developing a more efficient health care system. But the family may well have lost its entire savings, its home, and much of its income. That is not a modest cost.

So, who has the right to determine that treatment is inappropriate? Who has the right to make such decisions? The standard answer is clear. "Only the patient herself, at least within the options available to her in our health care system." Patient autonomy is still the supreme value we acknowledge in medical treatment decisions. That is one reason the SUPPORT study is so troubling: It suggests that patient autonomy is not upheld in the care of the terminally ill.

The SUPPORT study indicates that physicians are undermining patient autonomy by arrogating to themselves decisions that rightfully belong to the patient. But why should treatment decisions be restricted to the dyad? A genuine attempt to promote everyone's autonomy dictates that many treatment decisions should be family decisions. After all, that's the way people with families should make decisions that will dramatically alter the lives of members of their families. Medical decisions are no different. Sometimes, no doubt, family decisions are not possible, practical, or desirable. Even then, treatment decisions must attempt to maximize the autonomy of everyone whose life will be affected by the decision. If they do not, some people are inevitably marginalized or treated as a means merely.

Despite this argument, some may want to insist on preserving *patient* autonomy—the right of patients to make "their own" treatment decisions. After all, frightened and seriously ill people may not be able to hold their own in difficult and emotional family conversations. So, for practical reasons, it may be best to continue to let the patient decide.

But with autonomy comes responsibility. Indeed, the effects of our choices on the lives of others is the very cradle of moral responsibility. Thus, if we insist on patient autonomy, we must also insist that patients shoulder weighty moral responsibilities. We must learn to ask patients to consider not only what they want, but also the impact of their decisions on the lives of others. Often, what I want may not be a morally legitimate choice for me because it would impose burdens that are too great on others, particularly those who cannot easily refuse me.[2]

Thus, many competent patients like those in the SUPPORT study have not only a right to discuss treatment decisions with their physicians, they have an obligation to do so. They have not only a right, but a *duty* to fill out appropriate advance directives. And for many terminally ill patients, it is wrong to choose life-prolonging treatment, no matter how much they may want it. Often, it is even wrong not to choose, for that saddles the family with the burden and guilt of having to do so. An obligation to choose one's own death when one wants to live is a heavy obligation, indeed. But such may sometimes be the moral price of patient autonomy.

The physicians in the SUPPORT study have taken on the role of decision makers. It would be interesting to know why they have done so. One possibility is that they believe both patients and their families are incapable of making stable and responsible treatment decisions because both are in the throes of serious emotional crises. If family conferences are often not workable and patients should not be asked to bear the moral responsibility that comes with autonomy, perhaps decisions should be made by physicians after all.

Perhaps so. But not by physicians like those in the SUPPORT study. Not by *any* physicians who think of themselves as patient advocates, as most presumably still do. The role of patient advocacy may seem a noble one, but it is one-sided and unfair. It has seemed so self-evidently justified only because we have restricted our view to the traditional dyad. The advocacy stance is, in fact, one of the major reasons for the invisibility of families and their treatment as means to the patient's well-being. An ethic sufficiently sensitive to the patient's family would require physicians and other health care professionals to abandon the role of patient advocate. Or it would insist that they not make treatment decisions for patients with families. An advocate for one person is morally debarred from making decisions when more than one have legitimate interests at stake.

We must, then, move beyond the ethics of the dyad or even the contemporary triad. Instead, we must learn to think in terms of family justice. Fairness to all concerned will be a major factor in determining both who should decide and also what is the appropriate treatment at the end of life. That's the way decisions by and for people with families ought to be made—with everyone thinking about what will be best and fairest for all.

This idea might seem hopeless because families are so different and have such different conceptions of justice. We certainly have no theory of familial justice that is even remotely adequate. But questions of family justice cannot be legitimately avoided. Attempts to do so marginalize people. If families emerge from their invisibility, we will all be able to see many cases in which benefits to patients are not sufficient to justify the burdens they impose on their families. Ask yourself, Would you rather lose your career and all your savings at age 55, or lose a 50 percent chance of living an extra year with a terminal disease at age 83? Would anyone prefer the chance of an extra year?

But a health care system sensitive to the burdens treatment decisions impose on families is nowhere in sight. In fact, those who focus on the doctor–patient dyad will not even agree that such a system would be morally legitimate. In the foreseeable future, then, families will continue to be invisible, marginalized, or reduced to means. Costs will, no doubt, continue to be shifted to families. We will continue to be largely oblivious to the impact of our health care system and our treatment decisions on their lives.

In this context, the better the family—the more loyal, sensitive, and loving the caregivers within the family—the more we will take advantage of their resources and virtues. Unable or unwilling to divorce herself from her terrified and dying mother, Jane just keeps trying to hang in there. She and I have developed a little ritual. "How ya doing?" I ask when our paths cross. "I'm still vertical," Jane responds. "That's terrific, Jane, just terrific!" We smile sadly at the gallows humor. But the last time I saw her, she said, "If this goes on much longer, Mom is going to outlive *me.*"

NOTES

1. Kenneth E. Convinsky, et al., "The Impact of Serious Illness of Patients' Families," *Journal of the American Medical Association* 272 (1994):1839–44.

2. Many patients agree. There is beginning to be evidence that patients would prefer that life-prolonging treatment be discontinued when it has a serious financial impact on their family members. [See, for example, Ashwini Sehgal, et al., "How Strictly Do Dialysis Patients Want Their Advance Directives Followed?" *Journal of the American Medical Association* 267 (1992): 59–63.] But the interests of other family members do not have standing because the patient wants them considered; they have standing *whether or not* the patient wants to consider them.

Elder Abuse, Ethics, and Context

I. INTRODUCTION

For me, the pivotal moment in the conference on "Violence, Neglect, and the Elderly" came fairly early. I find myself returning over and over to a story that Margaret Hudson told to illustrate her claim that elder abuse is not always a bad person doing horrible things. Often, it is a good person stuck in an intolerable situation.

The story was about an elderly man struggling to care for his wife who was a victim of Alzheimer's. She had taken to wandering at night as well as during the day. As a result, she needed **constant** supervision—24 hours/day, 7 days/week. Her husband had no relief from this task; he was on the verge of physical collapse. One night in desperation he tied his wife to her bed. He then slept soundly for the first time in days and did not hear anything until she hit the floor.

A memorable story—it moved others in the audience, as well. But it was an aside in terms of Hudson's analysis. Her argument was not affected in any important way by her story; it is not even included in the written text of her talk.[1] She told the story only to make it clear that she is not insensitive to the problems facing caregivers who end up doing things that we might label abuse.

Still, we can wonder whether Hudson is sensitive enough. If she searches for a common meaning of the term "elder abuse" and in so doing effectively ignores the plight of caregivers, we can rightfully begin to wonder whether she is attentive enough to their problems. One wonders, for example, why the scenarios around which Hudson's research is organized say nothing about the situation of the caregivers and the impact that giving care makes on their own lives. Presumably, Hudson thinks that the situation of caregivers is irrelevant to what is or is not elder abuse. She invites all of us to think so, too.

Hudson is not alone in this; she is in the mainstream. The entire conference was well within the accepted paradigm in this respect. We all pretty much ignored the problems facing caregivers. We alluded to them from time to time, but our analyses were not importantly affected by concerns for abusive caregivers. Their problems were dismissed with an occasional aside that someone—the government, perhaps—should do something more to support those caring for the elderly.

It might seem perfectly appropriate that we ignored the situation of abusive caregivers—after all, we were gathered to advocate for victims of elder abuse, not for their abusers. But I will argue that we cannot get even so far as a definition of elder abuse without considering much more carefully the context in which the abuse occurs. The context must, of course, also be taken into consideration in proposing interventions into cases of possible elder abuse.

II. THE DEFINITION OF ABUSE AND THE SITUATION OF THE CAREGIVER

Is elder abuse wrong? That seems an odd question. Surely, if we can agree on nothing else, we can at least agree that elder abuse is bad, wrong, deplorable, and ought to stop. What could be clearer? The strangeness of the question—Is elder abuse wrong?—suggests that abuse (and neglect, as well) are inextricably moral notions. Other, equally strange statements point to the same conclusion. Do the following statements make sense? "Abusing his wife was the right thing to do in that situation." "Her obligation was clear and it was to neglect her mother." "His father was abused, but he was treated fairly."

The notions of elder abuse (and neglect) seem to rest squarely on the idea that the abused person has been wrongfully treated. Thus, too, the powerful feelings of revulsion when we contemplate the topic; we do not have similarly intense feelings of revulsion or outrage about old people in other harsh or unfortunate circumstances, no matter how harmful the result. But if the concept of abuse implies wrongful treatment, we cannot ascertain whether an elderly person is being abused until we know what is morally acceptable and what is wrongful treatment. We will first need an account of what the moral obligations of a caregiver to an elderly person are. Wrongful treatment occurs when moral obligations are not met.

Still, we may hesitate to embrace the conclusion that abuse is essentially a moral concept. Right and wrong, good and bad, moral and immoral are all very messy concepts. It is notoriously difficult to get agreement about moral concepts. If we hesitate, we might get some help from Thomas Murray.[2] During the final presentation of the conference, Murray distinguished three senses of "abuse" or "neglect"—the purely descriptive or objective, the moral, and the legal. If that distinction holds, we would be able to say that abuse **in the moral sense** is, indeed, an inextricably moral notion, but there is another, objective sense of abuse not dependent on moral notions.

But we cannot avoid the nasty problems of ethics by simply sticking to an objective definition. In the first place, we have just been wondering whether there really is a purely descriptive sense of a term like "abuse." But even if there is, it will not do the work we need. A purely descriptive or "objective" definition of elder abuse would be morally neutral; as such, it would not enable us to draw any conclusions about whether the activity so described is right or wrong, unjustified or perfectly appropriate. For that, we need a moral sense of the term.

The justification for legal intervention also rests on the moral definition of the term. Our strong sense of family privacy would shield a family from any intervention not wanted by all members of the family, unless someone is being wrongfully treated.

For these reasons, I will focus on the moral sense of elder abuse and elder neglect. I will cast my argument in terms of elder abuse, though it applies to elder neglect, as well. I will argue that elder abuse is a very contextual matter, heavily dependent on precisely what the conference ignored—the situation of the caregiver. Consequently, we need a very thick description of a case in order to tell whether or not something is elder abuse.

Let us return to Hudson's example. Is tying your demented wife to her bed elder abuse? That seems an easy question to answer. Of course! Surely any time anyone ties an elderly, demented person in her bed, it is elder abuse! Hudson also thinks it is clearly abuse—otherwise this narrative could not illustrate her point that people who abuse the elderly are often stuck in intolerable situations. I assume Hudson will find that most Americans agree.

But we still need to ask, what should the husband have done? Maybe he should have **handcuffed** her in bed. Would that have been better? With the 20/20 vision of hindsight, we might agree that it would have been. And it might have been better yet if he had used one of those restraints that many seem to believe should be entirely eliminated from nursing homes. Presumably, though, the husband had neither on hand—these are not common household tools. With the wisdom of hindsight, we might also think he should have anticipated this problem a month earlier, installed a lock on his wife's bedroom door, and **locked** her in her room each night when he went to bed.

Notice that we are tempted to call all of these alternatives elder abuse. Still, we cannot simultaneously recommend them to the husband and also say that they are elder abuse in the moral sense. If the most sensitive and humane option available to the husband was to restrain his demented wife in her bed or lock her in her room at night, then doing so cannot be elder abuse, not in the moral sense.

Now let us imagine a modified version of Hudson's case. The husband is a wealthy man. He can easily afford to hire round-the-clock care for his demented wife. He is well rested, for even if his wife becomes obstreperous in the middle of the night, it does not bother him—he sleeps in another wing of the house. Nevertheless, he ties his wife in her bed out of sheer malice or because he simply does not want to pay for someone to look after her. In **that** case, we have elder abuse. Given that scenario, what the husband did is clearly wrong and blameworthy.

Elder abuse in the moral sense can be identified only with the help of a thick description of the case, including many features of the situation of the caregiver. To ascertain whether an act is or is not elder abuse, we will need to know who cares for the "victim" and why, how long the caregiver has been providing care, what alternatives are available for giving care, what opportunities for relief the caregiver has, the physical and emotional reserves of this caregiver, the kinship relationship (if any) between caregiver and "victim," and much more.

It is worthwhile to pause here to note that the preceding arguments about the situation of the husband/caregiver can be extended to institutions and the paid caregivers who work in them. In his paper, Ben Rich pointed to many kinds of abuse of the elderly in nursing homes.[3] But I found elements of his discussion similarly unattuned to the situation of the caregivers. Granted, the situation of the staff of a nursing home is rarely even remotely as desperate as that of the husband in Hudson's story. If nothing else, you work your shift and then you can leave the whole situation.

Still, even in the setting of a nursing home, context is relevant to identifying elder abuse in the moral sense. If the demented residents of a nursing home are being sedated or physically restrained so that the staff can sit and gossip in the staff lounge, that is abuse. But if the staffing is very thin and there are so many things that must be attended to, perhaps restraining a resident or locking her in her room is the best, most fair, most humane thing the staff can do. I see no way to eliminate the situation of the caregivers—whether institutional or family—from a discussion of what elder abuse is.

The need to consider the situation of the caregivers reveals what I take to be a major difficulty in Hudson's research program. The scenarios she gives her respondents to test their intuitions about elder abuse are far too incomplete. Her respondents cannot or should not judge whether the activities she describes are abusive in any sense that is incompatible with their being the right thing to do. I suspect that what Hudson's respondents are doing is imaginatively filling in the needed details and then judging a much richer picture they have constructed, not simply the one-sentence description that Hudson has given them. When Hudson finds significant disagreement among her respondents, one major reason for this disagreement may well be that they are imagining different case scenarios. The agreement Hudson finds could also be spurious because people may be giving the same answer about what are really different imagined scenarios.

III. Principles for Contextualizing Obligation of Caregivers

Because the situation of the caregivers is relevant to judgments of abuse in the moral sense, we will not be able to come up with many, if any, actions which will **always** be elder abuse. (The only examples I can think of rest on a description of the action that is already pejorative, e.g., beating, drugging.) But it does not follow that there are no moral principles to help guide us in defining the moral concept of elder abuse. Some of these principles will be principles that point to morally relevant features of the caregiver's situation and her relationship to the elderly person she cares for.

It is these principles to which I wish to call attention. They tend to be forgotten. They certainly were forgotten at our conference. We tend to focus on the problems of dependent old people. When we do so, caregivers fade from view or are conceptualized as "problems" (abusers or neglecters), as "family support," or as "family resources" for providing care for an elderly person. This is especially true if we see ourselves as advocates for the elderly.

What, then, are the moral principles for defining a caregiver's obligations to the family member she cares for?

1. **Ought implies can**. No one is obligated to do more than she can. Consequently, the care an elderly person should receive from her caregiver depends on the caregiver's resource's—mental, emotional, physical, social, familial, and economic. However,

2. **Can does not imply ought**. No one is obligated, except for a very short time, to do "all they can" for someone else, not even for a member of her family. To think someone is so obligated is to treat that person as a mere means to the ends of that family member.

3. **Often, it is WRONG to do all you can for an elderly person, even if that is what you want to do**. Virtually everyone has other, conflicting obligations which must also be met. If nothing else, there are usually other family members whose needs and interests must be considered. Thus, a woman with children may well owe her mother less care than one who has no children; indeed, a woman who pays little attention to her children because she wants to give the best possible care to her mother is doing something wrong (even if she cannot be said to be abusing or neglecting them). Moreover, if an elderly person must be ignored, or even restricted or restrained so that time and attention can be devoted to fulfilling the caregiver's other obligations, it will sometimes be right to do so (providing other, more suitable alternatives are not available).

It may be possible to define a minimal level of care due to any member of one's family within the limits defined by these three principles. If there is enough food so that everyone can eat, old persons should be fed; if there is enough money to heat the house, an old person should also sleep in a heated room. But even this minimal level of care is conditioned by these three principles: If there is not enough for everyone to eat, it may be wrong to feed the elderly. Moreover, this is a minimal, even rudimentary level of care. Once a minimal level of care is being given, additional principles come into play to help determine whether a less minimalistic level of care is morally required.

4. **The wants and interests of caregivers are also relevant to defining the limits of their moral responsibilities to the elderly**. This follows from

the moral principle that no one is to be treated as a mere means for satisfying other people's ends. Thus, although "what is best for the elderly person" and "what the elderly person wants (or would have wanted)" are always relevant considerations, they are not by themselves sufficient to determine what should be done.[4] Family caregivers have lives of their own. Increases and decreases in the quality of life of the caregiver are just as important to moral judgment as changes in the quality of life of the dependent elderly. Appropriate care must be determined on the basis of fairness to all members of the family.[5]

Some have admitted that fairness to all is the appropriate standard when someone is being cared for at home, but they argue that the wishes or best interests of the patient are the standards for defining appropriate care in hospitals and other institutions.[6] But this is a deeply incoherent position: Hands dealt in the hospital often must be played out at home. In fact, harsh as it may sound, it could be right either to refuse to hospitalize an incompetent elderly person or to withdraw care from her in the hospital on the grounds that her continued existence is too burdensome for her family, especially her caregivers. To think otherwise is to reduce the caregiver to a means to the ends of the elderly person.

5. **What is owed to mentally competent elderly persons depends partly on how they act**. Competent elderly persons who act badly toward their family and/or caregivers merit less care, and care of lower quality, than those who behave well. In fact, an elderly person who behaves badly enough (in avoidable ways) may even merit her "abuse." Acknowledging this point is part and parcel of treating the elderly as morally capable persons: Any competent member of a family who regularly behaves badly enough toward the others merits less care from them. People, morally competent people, of any age can be nasty, mean, brutal, hateful, selfish, domineering, petty, vengeful, excessively demanding, etc. Members of their families rightfully may and often should take steps to protect themselves and their lives from such a person.

6. **What is owed to an elderly person, competent or incompetent, depends partly on how they treated others when they were younger, especially on how they treated those who now care for them**. A woman who, as a girl, was physically and sexually abused by her father certainly owes him much less when he becomes old than she would if he had been loving, generous, and supportive. Thus, not only the present situation, but also the history of relationships is relevant to defining the obligations of caregivers.

7. **Grossly imprudent earlier activity diminishes an elderly person's claim to assistance**. There is a bumper sticker that sometimes appears on the back of motor homes: "I'm spending my children's inheritance." While it may (or may not) be morally permissible to spend your children's inheritance, it is not permissible to spend lavishly and then come to them for financial assistance in your old age.

These, then, are a few of the moral principles that we must use to contextualize our accounts of elder abuse. Of course, such principles are not formulas which will enable us simply to read off the answer to questions about elder abuse. But they are considerations always to bear in mind when formulating judgments about cases of possible elder abuse.

IV. Social Abuse and Neglect of the Elderly

At this point, if not long before, some will want to object strongly: "Any demented woman who is locked in her room or tied in her bed **is** being abused! Only she is being abused by **society**, not by her caregiver. Perhaps her husband is being abused by society, as well."

"After all," the objection continues, "if appropriate social services were in place, this old couple would not be in such a desperate situation and there would be no need and no temptation to tie the wife to her bed. Recognizing the responsibility of society for its elderly citizens would allow us to identify cases of elder abuse in the moral sense without examining the situation of the caregiver. It is **social** abuse of the elderly that Hudson's story illustrates."

Our conference dealt largely with elder abuse on an "up close and personal" level. That seems to make sense, since abuse requires an abuser, presumably some specifiable individual. It also makes sense if our goal is to identify specific activities that constitute elder abuse, or if we are wondering whether or not to intervene in a particular situation.

But the individual level is also the level on which we Americans are most comfortable with moral analysis. Social responsibility or community obligations do not get very far with us. This preference for individual responsibility can easily slide into a kind of moral isolationism: "I'll take care of me and mine; you worry about you and yours."

Such moral isolationism would leave us with insoluble problems about dependent elderly people who have no children, no surviving children, or children who either simply cannot or will not care for their parents. If we do not think it appropriate for elderly people with limited financial resources and no family caregivers simply to be left to die in the streets or in their apartments, such moral isolationism cannot be justified.

If moral isolationism cannot be justified, and if we nonetheless wish to keep our moral discussion on the level of individual responsibility, we need to learn to ask: What do we individually owe to old people who are not part of our families or personal friends? We also need to ask this question whenever our social institutions fail to meet their responsibilities to the elderly.

I cannot even begin here to give an account of the social obligations to the elderly, but a few basic points will suffice to show that the notion of social responsibility to the elderly must also be contextualized.

1. **In order to generate a theory of elder abuse by society, we will need a theory of what a society such as ours owes its older people**. "A society such as ours"—social responsibility is thus contextualized from the very beginning, as wealthy societies owe their elderly much more than societies that exist on the margin of subsistence.

Even in a wealthy society such as ours, this theory of social responsibility cannot simply be a litany of what old people need. Just because someone has an unmet need, it does not follow that society has an obligation to meet that need. There may be some needs, e.g., the need for individual affirmation or personal care, that just cannot be met by any society. In addition, it may be impossible to meet everyone's needs, as satisfying one person's needs is incompatible with satisfying the needs of others. For example, a frail, terrified, old man may need his daughter around at all times, but she needs time to herself.

What is more, there are other Americans who have needs every bit as pressing as those of the elderly. Thus, huge questions of intergenerational justice will have to be addressed. For example, old people get better health care than children in this country, and it is arguable that they get better health care than working people, as well. Is that just? We provide nursing home care for elderly people who have nowhere else to go. We do not, however, provide a shelter of even remotely comparable quality for homeless people, including homeless children. Is that just?

2. We will also need a theory of what ought to be done if a society is not going to meet its obligations to all its members. We face a burgeoning taxpayer revolt in this country. In this context, it may well be that our society simply will not meet its theoretical obligations to all its members in need, either through public or private assistance. We citizens of the United States simply may not feel the obligations which a theory of justice to the elderly states that we have.

Where there are severe budgetary constraints, should we provide decent shelter for all Americans before we provide nursing home care for the demented elderly? Is hunger in children less morally justifiable than hunger in the elderly? Should we provide basic health care for all Americans before we contemplate transferring elderly people to hospitals for expensive, high-tech care? Answers to questions like these are what policy makers most need, not an account of what a wealthy society theoretically owes each of its citizens.

Thus, even the concept of **social** abuse of the elderly has to be contextualized. In the setting of the United States in the 1990s, we might argue that American voters are abusing the elderly. However theoretically sound such an argument might be, it does not seem likely to get very far. Alternatively, we might argue that politicians who divide up the tax money ought to have been more generous with funding social programs for older people, but it is far from clear that that is true.

Still, even if such arguments were successful, they show only that our social situation should be different. They do not tell us what should be done for old people **in our situation.** Answers to the question of what social agencies should do **in our situation** might throw the couple in Hudson's example back on their own resources. Given our limited social will to help others in need, it may well be that we ought not to devote the available resources to nursing home care for this man's demented wife or even to temporary relief for him.

Thus, we again face the very real possibility that the demented wife is not being abused. Given limited funding, social institutions ought not assume care of this demented woman. So, given the context, this couple is not a victim of social abuse in the moral sense . . . unless perhaps by American voters. Since her husband is providing the best care he can for this woman, she is not being abused in the moral sense by him, either.

V. ABUSE, INTERVENTION, AND CONTEXT

Increased attention to the situation and interests of caregivers could, I think, yield genuine benefits. I turn now to a few practical implications of a more contextualized discussion of elder abuse.

1. **We must sharply distinguish abuse in the moral sense from virtually any list of abusive activities**. There will be only an **extremely** short list, if any at all, of activities which are always abusive. The fact that an elderly person is physically pushed into her room and locked there, physically restrained, threatened with physical harm, shouted at and frightened, or even hit does not necessarily mean that she is abused. To find out whether she is abused, we must know much more about the situation.

2. We **must also recognize that "abusive activities" are not necessarily signs that genuine care or concern is lacking**. Since many apparently abusive activities are not abuse in the moral sense, these activities do not necessarily reflect badly on the intentions or character of the caregiver. Blame and accusations will, in such cases, be inappropriate. Moreover, even if something genuinely is abuse (in the moral sense), it may be that the caregiver should be **excused** for what she did. We all experience lapses from good behavior even within contexts of genuine care—when we are angry, fatigued, harried or rushed, depressed, or simply frustrated due to lack of time to do what **we** want. Like the rest of us, caregivers will occasionally do things that are wrong, but for which they should be excused.

Where genuine care is present, it may be possible to help the caregiver to reform or to "do better." But we must also recognize that attempts to get caregivers to reform or to do better may be misguided. The husband in Hudson's story got into trouble because he was already trying to do too much for his wife. But even more important for our purposes, "doing better" would often only require even more heroic sacrifices on the part of caregivers; and that might well mean that their legitimate interests would be even more dramatically short-changed. When this is the case, it may be wrong even to suggest that the caregiver try to do better. Such suggestions may be rightfully resented.

3. **If we are to respond effectively to the plight of those who seem to be victims of elder abuse, we must, paradoxically, stop focusing exclu-**

sively on harm to them. We must also consider the situation of the care-givers. If we can get some relief for the husband in Hudson's story, it will translate into better conditions for his wife, assuming he still genuinely cares for her. If we cannot get relief for him, no amount of investigation and intervention short of removing her from her home will help her much in the long run.

4. **An "abusive" situation may be the best situation available for an elderly person, even if it is occasionally genuinely abusive**. Removing "abused" old persons from their abusive environments may be contrary to their interests. If a husband still genuinely cares for his wife, then continuing to live with him may be the best alternative for her, even if she is "abused." After all, he is familiar with her particular desires and emotional responses. For this reason, he may be both willing and able to respond more appropriately to those needs. In their home, he is also much more likely to be there when she needs him than if he must visit her in an institution. For that matter, their home is where she feels at home. Finally, there is genuine personal affirmation in being cared for by those who love us, even if they are sometimes abusive, rather than by paid strangers. In fact, an abusive situation may be the best situation for an old person even in cases that involve physical abuse and the risk of serious bodily injury.

This observation was recently corroborated by a social worker who reported that fear of being removed from their homes is one of the primary reasons elderly people do not report abuse.[7] If she is correct, many old people believe they are better off where they are, their abuse notwithstanding. Moreover, if—as seems likely—social funding for alternatives to home care becomes more skimpy and families must shoulder even more of the burdens of long-term care of the elderly, there will be more and more cases in which an abusive situation is the best available situation for an old person. We must face the fact that this is one of the consequences of our declining willingness to provide a social safety net for people, including the elderly.

5. **Since an abusive situation may be the best situation for an elderly person, intervention may be unwarranted in cases of abuse**. Attempts to empower an old person so that **she** will request intervention may also be misguided. We must face the fact that an elderly person may not be requesting intervention because she quite correctly believes her present situation, abusive though it be, is the best available situation for her. Intervention may thus be paternalism gone awry—paternalism that does

not even manage to promote the best interests of the victim. When the abusive situation is the best situation for an old person, if no intervention seems likely to improve that situation, none is warranted.

6. **On the policy level, we must break the conceptual connection between intervention and abuse (or neglect)**. In many situations, applying the concepts of abuse and neglect will actually be counterproductive. Abuse and neglect are accusations. Good people caught in intolerable situations rightly resent such labels. Those caring for the elderly often need assistance, and we must find ways to help them without resorting to the rationale that we are intervening to protect the elderly from abuse.

7. **Those working in social agencies must not see themselves as advocates for the elderly victims**. We must not focus only on harm to the victim of abuse even if our ultimate aim is to help the abused. More basically, our ultimate aim ought not to be simply helping the abused. Instead, those dealing with elder abuse must be sensitive to the needs and interests of **all** involved, fair-minded about what is reasonable to expect of caregivers in their particular situations, and genuinely interested in designing interventions that would improve the lives of **all** members of the family. If family caregivers recognized that they and their families were being approached in this fair-minded way, there would be much less resistance to intervention. Indeed, intervention would then normally be welcomed by caregivers as long-sought, much needed assistance.

8. **All of the above notwithstanding, there remain genuine cases of inexcusable elder abuse (in the moral sense). Often, even criminal prosecution will be part of the appropriate intervention**. Although my purpose in this paper has been to call attention to a badly neglected "other side of the story," I certainly do not deny that there are also many cases of elder abuse in the moral sense. Caregivers are not all good people stuck in intolerable situations. The variation among caregivers is immense—caregivers (and the elderly) are just about as good and as bad as the rest of us. That is part of the reason we need a contextual account of "elder abuse." Intervention, too, must be tailor-made to the specific situation. Consequently, appropriate intervention cannot always be designed and justified by the one, simple rationale that intervention is needed to stop elder abuse or neglect.

In sum, we need richer, subtler, more contextual (and more complicated!) thinking and policies about "elder abuse." Both in our thinking and in our interventions, we need to contextualize—to consider the situation and intentions of the caregiver, the relationship (including the history of the relationship) between the elderly person and her caregiver, the situation they share, the available alternatives, and much, much more.

A contextualized account is a theoretically more sound account both of what caregivers owe the elderly and of what elder abuse is. It also yields important practical benefits. We must not only sensitize ourselves to the situation of caregivers, but also generate ethical analyses that adequately reflect such sensitivity. We must begin to think in terms of what is fair to all, rather than simply what is best, or merely not harmful, for the elderly. Though the stance of an advocate for the "abused" elderly may seem a noble stance, morally adequate analyses or plans for intervention cannot be generated from an advocacy standpoint. Advocacy in such situations implicitly reduces caregivers to mere means to the ends of the elderly and often one-sidedly misdescribes the moral situation. It also tends to obscure appropriate interventions. All are morally unacceptable.

NOTES

1. M. Hudson. "Expert and Public Perspectives in Defining Elder Abuse and Neglect." *Violence, Neglect, and the Elderly*. Ed. R. B. Edwards & E. E. Bittar. Greenwich, CT. JAI Press; 1996. (pp. 1–21).

2. Murray, T. "Ethical Obligations to the Elderly in a Changing Society." Advances in Bioethics, *Violence, Neglect, and the Elderly*. Ed. R. B. Edwards & E. E. Bittar. Greenwich, CT. JAI Press; 1996. (pp. 139–154).

3. B. Rich. "Elements Compromising the Autonomy of the Elderly." *Violence, Neglect, and the Elderly*. Ed. Edwards, R. B. & Bittar, E. E. Greenwich, CT. JAI Press; 1996. (pp. 57–90).

4. J. Hardwig. "What About the Family?—The Role of Family Interests in Medical Decision Making." *Hastings Center Report* 20 (1990): 5–10.

5. J. Hardwig. "The problem of Proxies with Interests of Their Own—Toward a Better Theory of Proxy Decisions." *Journal of Clinical Ethics* 4 (1993): 20–27.

6. B. Collopy, N. Dubler, and C. Zuckerman. "The Ethics of Home Care: Autonomy and Accommodation." *Hastings Center Report 20*, special supplement (1990): 1–16.

7. National Public Radio. Morning Edition 5/16/95.

Dying at the Right Time

Reflections on (Un)assisted Suicide

Let us begin with two observations about chronic illness and death:

1. Death does not always come at the right time. We are all aware of the tragedies involved when death comes too soon. We are afraid that it might come too soon for us. By contrast, we may sometimes be tempted to deny that death can come too late—wouldn't everyone want to live longer? But in our more sober moments, most of us know perfectly well that death can come too late.

2. Discussions of death and dying usually proceed as if death came only to hermits—or others who are all alone. But most of the time, death is a death in the family. We are connected to family and loved ones. We are sustained by these connections. They are a major part of what makes life worth living for most of us.

Because of these connections, when death comes too soon, the tragedy is often twofold: a tragedy both for the person who is now dead and for those of us to whom she was connected. We grieve both for our loved one who is gone and for ourselves who have lost her. On one hand, there is the unrealized good that life would have been for the dead person herself—what she could have become, what she could have experienced, what she wanted for herself. On the other, there is the contribution she would have made to others and the ways *their* lives would have been enriched by her.

We are less familiar with the idea that death can come too late. But here, too, the tragedy can be twofold. Death can come too late because of what living on means to the person herself. There are times when someone does not (or would not) want to live like this, times when she believes she would be better off dead. At times like these, suicide or assisted suicide becomes a perfectly rational choice, perhaps even the best available option for her. We are then forced to ask, "Does someone have a right to die?" Assisted suicide may then be an act of compassion, no more than relieving her misery.

There are also, sadly, times when death comes too late because *others*—family and loved ones—would be better off if someone were dead. (Better off overall, despite the loss of a loved one.) Since lives are deeply intertwined, the lives of the rest of the family can be dragged down, impoverished, compromised, perhaps even ruined because of what they must go through if she lives on. When death comes too late because of the effect of someone's life on her loved ones, we are, I think, forced to ask, "Can someone have a duty to die?" Suicide may then be an attempt to do what is right; it may be the only loving thing to do. Assisted suicide would then be helping someone do the right thing.

Most professional ethicists—philosophers, theologians, and bioethicists—react with horror at the very idea of a duty to die. Many of them even argue that euthanasia and physician-assisted suicide should not be legalized because then some people might somehow get the idea that they have a duty to die. To this way of thinking, someone who got that idea could only be the victim of vicious social pressure or perverse moral reasoning. But when I ask my classes for examples of times when death would come too late, one of the first conditions students always mention is: "when I become a burden to my family." I think there is more moral wisdom here than in the dismay of these ethicists.

Death does not always come at the right time. I believe there are conditions under which I would prefer not to live, situations in which I would be better off dead. But I am also absolutely convinced that I may one day face a duty or responsibility to die. In fact, as I will explain later, I think many of us will one day have this duty.

To my way of thinking, the really serious questions relating to euthanasia and assisted suicide are: Who would be better off dead? Who has a duty to die. *When* is the right time to die? And if my life should be over, who should kill me?[1] However, I know that others find much of what I have said here surprising, shocking, even morally offensive. So before turning to these questions that I want us to think about, I need to explain why I think someone can be better off dead and why someone can have a duty to die. (The explanation of the latter will have to be longer, since it is by far the less familiar and more controversial idea.)

WHEN SOMEONE WOULD BE BETTER OFF DEAD

Others have discussed euthanasia or physician-assisted suicide when the patient would be better off dead.[2] Here I wish to emphasize two points often omitted from discussion: (1) Unrelieved pain is not the only reason someone would be better off dead. (2) Someone can be better off dead even if she has no terminal illness.

1. If we think about it for even a little while, most of us can come up with a list of conditions under which we believe we would rather be dead than continue to live. Severe and unrelieved pain is one item on that list. Permanent unconsciousness may be another. Dementia so severe that we no longer recognize ourselves or our loved ones is yet another. There are some people who prefer not to live with quadriplegia. A future shaped by severe deterioration (such as that which accompanies MS, ALS, AIDS, or Huntington's chorea) is a future that some people prefer not to live out.

(Our lists would be different because our lives and values are different. The fact that some people would not or do not want to live with quadriplegia or AIDS, for example, does not mean that others should not want to live like that, much less that their lives are not worth living. That is very important. The point here is that almost all of us can make a list of conditions under which we would rather not live, and that uncontrolled pain is not the only item on most of our lists.)

Focusing the discussion of euthanasia and assisted suicide on pain ignores the many other varieties of suffering that often accompany chronic illness and dying: dehumanization, loss of independence, loss of control, a sense of meaninglessness or purposelessness, loss of mental capabilities, loss of mobility, disorientation and confusion, sorrow over the impact of one's illness and death on one's family, loss of ability even to recognize loved ones, and more. Often, these causes of suffering are compounded by the awareness that the future will be even bleaker. Unrelieved pain is simply not the only condition under which death is preferable to life, nor the only legitimate reason for a desire to end one's life.

2. In cases of terminal illness, death eventually offers the dying person relief from all her suffering. Consequently, things can be even

worse when there is NO terminal illness, for then there is no end in sight. Both pain and suffering are often much worse when they are not accompanied by a terminal illness. People with progressive dementia, for example, often suffer much more if they are otherwise quite healthy. I personally know several old people who would be delighted to learn that they have a terminal illness. They feel they have lived long enough—long enough to have outlived all their loved ones and all sense of a purpose for living. For them, even daily existence is much worse because there is no end in sight.

Discussions of euthanasia and physician-assisted suicide cannot, then, be restricted to those with unrelieved pain and terminal illness. We must also consider requests made by those who have no untreatable pain and no terminal illness. Often, their case for relief is even more compelling.

Sometimes, a refusal of medical treatment will be enough to bring relief. Competent adults who are suffering from an illness have a well-established moral and legal right to decline any form of medical treatment, including life-prolonging medical treatment. Family members who must make medical decisions for incompetent people also have the right to refuse any form of medical treatment on their behalf, so long as they are acting in accordance with the known wishes or best interests of their loved one. No form of medical treatment is compulsory when someone would be better off dead.[3]

But those who would be better off dead do not always have terminal illnesses; they will not always need any form of medical treatment, not even medically supplied food and water. The right to refuse medical treatment will not help these people. Moreover, death due to untreated illness can be agonizingly slow, dehumanizing, painful, and very costly, both in financial and emotional terms. It is often very hard. Refusing medical treatment simply will not always ensure a dignified, peaceful, timely death. We would not be having a national debate about physician-assisted suicide and euthanasia if refusal of medical treatment were always enough to lead to a reasonably good death. When death comes too late, we may need to do more than refuse medical treatment.

RELIGION AND ENDING A LIFE

Some people can easily see that there are people who would be better off dead. But they still cannot accept suicide or physician-assisted suicide because they believe we have a duty to God not to take our own lives. For them, human life is a gift from God and it remains a gift no matter how much pain and suffering it may bring. It is a sin or an offense against God, the giver of life, to take your own life or to help someone else end theirs. Such believers may also feel that no one should be allowed to end their lives—every life is a gift from God, even the lives of those who do not believe that this is so.

I do not understand this position for two reasons. First, it involves the assumption that it is possible to take a human life (our own or someone else's) *before* God wants it ended, but we cannot possibly preserve it *after* God wants it ended. For if we do not make that assumption, we face *two* dangers—the danger that we are prolonging human life beyond its divine purpose, as well as the danger that we are ending it too soon. If we can extend life longer than God intends, suicide and physician-assisted suicide may be more in accord with God's wishes than attempts to preserve that life.

I can understand the view that everyone dies at precisely the right time, the moment God intends. If that is so, people who commit suicide or who are intentionally killed by physicians also die at precisely the moment God wants them to die. I can also understand the view that we can take life before God wants it ended but we can also extend life longer than God wants it prolonged. But I cannot make sense of the view that we can end a human life too soon but not preserve it too long. Surely, God has given us both abilities or neither one.

I also have a second difficulty with this religious objection to suicide, assisted suicide, and euthanasia. Suppose there is a right time to die, a divinely ordained moment when God wants each life to end. Even so, we have no right to assume that God will "take my life" when it's the right time for me to die. In fact, we cannot even assume that God will send a terminal illness that will kill me at the right time. There could be a religious test—God may want me to take my own life and the question is whether I will meet this final challenge. Or a God who loves me might see that I would benefit spiritually from the process of coming to the conclusion that I should end my own life and then preparing to take it. That might be a fitting ending for me, the culminating step in my spiritual growth or development.

In short, a God not totally obsessed with the sheer quantity of our lives may well have purposes for us that are incompatible with longer life—even if we want to live longer. So, I think we should not believe that we always have a duty to God not to take our lives or to assist others in ending theirs. God may want me to step up and assume the responsibility for ending my own life or for seeing that someone else's suffering is ended. This observation leads to our next question: Can there be a responsibility or duty to die?

THE DUTY TO DIE

I may well one day have a duty to die, a duty most likely to arise out of my connections with my family and loved ones.[4] Sometimes preserving my life can only devastate the lives of those who care about me. I do not believe I am idiosyncratic, morbid, or morally perverse in believing this. I am trying to take steps to prepare myself mentally and spiritually to make sure that I will be able to take my life if I should one day have such a duty. I need to prepare myself; it might be a very difficult thing for me to do.

Our individualistic fantasy about ourselves sometimes leads us to imagine that lives are separate and unconnected, or that they could be so if we chose. If lives were unconnected, then things that happen in my life would not or need not affect others. And if others were not (much) affected by my life, I would have no duty to consider the impact of my life on others. I would then be morally free to choose whatever life and death I prefer for myself. I certainly would have no duty to die when I would prefer to live.

Most discussions of assisted suicide and euthanasia implicitly share this individualistic fantasy: They just ignore the fact that people are connected and lives intertwined. As a result, they approach issues of life or death as if the only person affected is the one who lives or dies. They mistakenly assume the pivotal issue is simply whether the person *herself* prefers not to live like this and whether *she herself* would be better off dead.[5]

But this is morally obtuse. The fact is we are not a race of hermits—most of us are connected to family and loved ones. We prefer it that way. We would not want to be all alone, especially when we are seriously ill, as we age, and when we are dying. But being with others is not all benefits and pleasures; it brings responsibilities, as well. For then what happens to us and the choices we make can dramatically affect the lives of our loved ones. It is these connections that can, tragically, generate obligations to die, as continuing to live takes too much of a toll on the lives of those connected to us.[6]

The lives of our loved ones can, we know, be seriously compromised by caring for us. The burdens of providing care or even just supervision 24 hours a day, 7 days a week, are often overwhelming.[7] But it can also be emotionally devastating simply to be married to a spouse who is increasingly distant, uncommunicative, unresponsive, foreign, and unreachable. A local newspaper tells the story of a woman with Alzheimer's who came running into her den screaming: "That man's trying to have sex with me! He's trying to have sex with me! Who IS that man?!" That man was her loving husband of more than 40 years who had devoted the past 10 years of his life to caring for her (Smith, 1995). How terrible that experience must have been for her. But how terrible those years must be for him, too.

We must also acknowledge that the lives of our loved ones can also be devastated just by having to *pay* for health care for us. A recent study documented the financial aspects of caring for a dying member of a family. Only those who had illnesses severe enough to give them less than a 50 percent chance to live 6 more months were included in this study. When these patients survived their initial hospitalization and were discharged, about one-third required considerable caregiving from their families; in 20 percent of cases a family member had to quit work or make some other major lifestyle change; almost one-third of these families lost all of their savings, and just under 30 percent lost a major source of income (Covinski et al., 1994).

A chronic illness or debilitating injury in a family is a misfortune. It is, most often, nobody's fault; no one is responsible for this illness or injury. But then we face choices about how we will respond to this misfortune. That is where the responsibility comes in and fault can arise. Those of us with families and loved ones always have a responsibility not to make selfish or self-centered decisions about our lives. We should not do just what we want or just what is best for *us*. Often, we should choose in light of what is best for all concerned.

Our families and loved ones have obligations to stand by us and to support us through debilitating illness and death. They must be prepared to make sacrifices to respond to an illness in the family. We are well aware of this responsibility and most families meet it rather well. In fact, families deliver more than 80 percent of the long-term care in the US, almost always at great personal cost.

But responsibility in a family is not a one-way street. When we become seriously ill or debilitated, we too may have to make sacrifices. There are limits to what we can ask our loved ones to do to support us, even in sickness. There are limits to what they should be prepared to do for us—only rarely and for a limited period of time should they do all they can for us.

Somehow we forget that sick, infirm, and dying adults also have obligations to their families and loved ones: a responsibility, for example, to try to protect the lives of loved ones from serious threats or greatly impoverished quality, or an obligation to avoid making choices that will jeopardize or seriously compromise their futures. Our obligations to our loved ones must be taken into consideration in making decisions about the end of life. It is out of these responsibilities that a duty to die can develop.

Tragically, sometimes the best thing you can do for your loved ones is to remove yourself from their lives. And the only way you can do that may be to remove yourself from existence. This is not a happy thought. Yet we must recognize that suicides and requests for assisted suicide may be motivated by love. Sometimes, it's simply the only loving thing to do.

WHO HAS A DUTY TO DIE?

Sometimes it is clear when someone has a duty to die. But more often, not. *WHO* has a duty to die? And *WHEN*–under what conditions? To my mind, these are right questions, the questions we should be asking. Many of us may one day badly need answers to just these questions.

But I cannot supply answers here, for two reasons. In the first place, answers will have to be very particular and individualized . . . to the person, to the situation of her family, to the relationships within the family, etc. There will not be simple answers that apply to everyone.

Secondly and perhaps even more importantly, those of us with family and loved ones should not define our duties unilaterally. Especially not a decision about a duty to die. It would be isolating and distance-creating for me to decide without consulting them what is too much of a burden for my loved ones to bear. That way of deciding about my moral duties is not only atomistic, it also treats my family and loved ones paternalistically-*THEY* must be allowed to speak for themselves about the burdens my life imposes on them and how they feel about bearing those burdens.

I believe in family decision making. Important decisions for those whose lives are interwoven should be made *together*, in a family discussion. Granted, a conversation about whether I have a duty to die would often be a tremendously difficult conversation. The temptations to be dishonest in such conversations could be enormous. Nevertheless, if we can, we should have just such an agonizing discussion—partly because it will act as a check on the information, perceptions, and reasoning of all of us; but perhaps even more importantly, because it affirms our connectedness at a critical juncture in our lives. Honest talk about difficult matters almost always strengthens relationships.

But many families seem to be unable to talk about death at all, much less a duty to die. Certainly most families could not have this discussion all at once, in one sitting. It might well take a number of discussions to be able to approach this topic. But even if talking about death is impossible, there are always behavioral clues—about your caregiver's tiredness, physical condition, health, prevailing mood, anxiety, outlook, overall well-being, etc. And families unable to talk about death can often talk about those clues. There can be conversations about how the caregiver is feeling, about finances, about tensions within the family resulting from the illness, about concerns for the future. Deciding whether you have a duty to die based on these behavioral clues and conversation about them is more relational than deciding on your own about how burdensome this relationship and care must be.[8]

For these two reasons, I cannot say when someone has a duty to die. But I can suggest a few ideas for discussion of this question. I present them here without much elaboration or explanation.

1. There is more duty to die when prolonging your life will impose greater burdens—emotional burdens, caregiving, disruption of life plans, and, yes, financial hardship—on your family and loved ones. This is the fundamental insight underlying a duty to die.

2. There is greater duty to die if your loved ones' lives have already been difficult or impoverished (not just financially)—if they have had only a small share of the good things that life has to offer.

3. There is more duty to die to the extent that your loved ones have already made great contributions—perhaps even sacrifices—to make your life a good one. Especially if you have not made similar sacrifices for their well-being.

4. There is more duty to die to the extent that you have already lived a full and rich life. You have already had a full share of the good things life offers.

5. Even if you have not lived a full and rich life, there is more duty to die as you grow older. As we become older, there is a diminishing chance that we will be able to make the changes that would now be required to turn our lives around. As we age, we will also be giving up less by giving up our lives, if only because we will sacrifice fewer years of life.

6. There is less duty to die to the extent that you can make a good adjustment to your illness or handicapping condition, for a good adjustment means that smaller sacrifice will be required of loved ones and there is more compensating interaction for them. (However, we must also recognize that some diseases—Alzheimer's or Huntington's chorea—will eventually take their toll on your loved ones no matter how courageously, resolutely, even cheerfully you manage to face that illness.)

7. There is more duty to die to the extent that the part of you that is loved will soon be gone or seriously compromised. There is also more duty to die when you are no longer capable of giving love. Part of the horror of Alzheimer's or Huntington's, again, is that it destroys the person we loved, leaving a stranger and eventually only a shell behind. By contrast, someone can be seriously debilitated and yet clearly still the person we love.

In an old person, "I am not ready to die yet" does not excuse one from a duty to die. To have reached the age of, say, 80 years without being ready to die is itself a moral failing, the sign of a life out of touch with life's basic realities.

A duty to die seems very harsh, and sometimes it is. But if I really do care for my family, a duty to protect their lives will often be accompanied by a deep desire to do so. I will normally want to protect those I love. This is not only my duty, it is also my desire. In fact, I can easily imagine wanting to spare my loved ones the burden of my existence more than I want anything else.

If I Should Be Dead, Who Should Kill Me?

We need to reframe our discussions of euthanasia and physician-assisted suicide. For we must recognize that pleas for assisted suicide are sometimes requests for relief from pain and suffering, sometimes requests for help in fulfilling one's obligations, and sometimes both. If I should be dead for either of these reasons, who should kill me?

Like a responsible life, a responsible death requires that we think about our choices in the context of the web of relationships of love and care that surround us. We must be sensitive to the suffering as well as the joys we cause others, to the hardships as well as the benefits we create for them. So, when we ask, "Who should kill me?", we must remember that we are asking for a death that will reduce the suffering of *both* me and my family as much as possible. We are searching for the best ending, not only for me, but for *everyone concerned*—in the preparation for death, the moment of death, and afterwards, in the memory and ongoing lives of loved ones and family.

Although we could perhaps define a new profession to assist in suicides—euthanasians—there are now really only three answers to the question, "Who should kill me?" (1) I should kill myself. (2) A loved one or family member should kill me. (3) A physician should kill me. I will consider these three possibilities. I will call these *unassisted* suicide, *family*-assisted suicide, and *physician*-assisted suicide.

(1) Unassisted suicide: I should kill myself

The basic intuition here is that each of us should take responsibility for herself. I am primarily the one who wants relief from my pain and suffering, or it is fundamentally my own duty to die and *I* should be the one to do my duty. Moreover, intentionally ending a life is a very messy business—a heavy, difficult thing for anyone to have to do. If possible, I should not drag others into it. Often, I think, this is the right idea—I should be the one to kill myself.

But not always. We must remember that some people are physically unable to do so—they are too weak or incapacitated to commit suicide without assistance. Less persuasive perhaps are those who just can't bring themselves to do it. Without the assistance of someone, many lack the know-how or means to end their lives in a peaceful, dignified fashion. Finally, many attempted suicides—even serious attempts at suicide—fail or result in terrible deaths. Those who have worked in hospitals are familiar with suicide attempts that leave people with permanent brain damage or their faces shot off. There are also fairly common stories of people eating their own vomit after throwing up the medicine they hoped would end their lives.

Even more importantly, if I must be the one to kill myself, that may force me to take my life earlier than would otherwise be necessary. I cannot wait until I become physically debilitated or mentally incompetent, for then it will be too late for me to kill myself. I might be able to live quite comfortably for a couple more years, if I could count on someone else to take my life later. But if I cannot count on help from anyone, I will feel pressure to kill myself when unavoidable suffering for myself or my loved ones appears on the horizon, instead of waiting until it actually arrives.

Finally, many suicides are isolating—I can't die with my loved ones around me if I am planning to use carbon monoxide from automobile exhaust to end my life. For most of us, a meaningful end of life requires an affirmation of our connection with loved ones and so we do not want to die alone.

The social taboo against ending your own life promotes another type of isolation. The secrecy preceding many suicides creates conditions for misunderstanding or lack of understanding on the part of loved ones—Why did she do it? Why didn't I see that she was going to kill herself? Why didn't I do something to help? Secrecy and lack of understanding often compound the suffering family and loved ones go through when someone ends their life.

Unassisted suicide—I should kill myself—is not always the answer. Perhaps, then, my loved ones should participate in ending my life.

(2) Family-assisted suicide: A member of my family should kill me

At times, we may have a moral obligation to help others end their lives, especially those close to us, those we love. I can easily imagine myself having an obligation to help a loved one end her life and I hope my family will come to my assistance if my death does not come at the right time. What should be the role of family and loved ones in ending a life?

They might help me get information about reliable and peaceful methods for ending my life. They might also be able to help me get the drugs I need, if that is the method I choose. Like most people, I would also very much want my loved ones to participate, at least to the extent of being there with me when I die.

For reasons already mentioned, I would hope I could talk over my plans with my loved ones, both to reassure myself and check on my reasoning, and also to help them work through some of the emotional reaction to my death. Some people believe that families should not be involved in decisions about the end of life because they are in the grips of powerful emotions that lead to wildly inappropriate decisions. (A familiar example is the difficulty many families have in deciding to withdraw medical treatment even when their loved one is clearly dying.) Families will always be gripped by powerful emotions over a death in the family. But appropriate decisions are not necessarily unemotional or uninvolved decisions. And I think inappropriate reactions or decisions stem largely from lack of the discussions I advocate or from an attempt to compress them into one, brief, pressure-packed conversation, often in the uncomfortable setting of a hospital.

So, a good death for all concerned would usually involve my family—the preparation for taking my life, at least, would be family-assisted. My loved ones should know; they should, if possible, understand. They should not be surprised. Hopefully my loved ones could come to agree with my decision. They should have had time to come to terms with the fact that I plan to end my life. Indeed, I should have helped them begin to deal emotionally with my death. All that would help to ease their suffering and also my concern about how my death will affect them. It would reaffirm our connectedness. It would also comfort me greatly to feel that I am understood and known by my loved ones as I take this important step.

More than this I cannot ask of them, for two related reasons. The first is that actually killing a loved one would usually be extremely difficult. It would be a searing and unforgettable experience that could well prove very hard to live with afterwards. Killing a loved one at her request *might* leave you feeling relieved—it could give you the satisfaction of feeling you had done what needed to be done. In cases of extreme debility or great suffering, family-assisted suicide might be experienced as a loving act of kindness, compassion, and mercy. It would still be very hard. Much harder would be killing me because I have a duty to die, a duty to die because my life is too great a burden *for the one who now must kill me*. I cannot ask that of someone I love. I fear that they would suffer too much from taking my life.

I might be wrong about this, however. It might be that, though difficult indeed, being killed lovingly and with your consent by your spouse or your child would be a final testimonial to a solid, trusting, and caring relationship. There might be no more powerful reaffirmation of the strength of your relationship, even in the face of death. The traumatic experience for the family members who assist in the suicide might be a healing experience for them, as well. We know so little about family-assisted suicide.

But in any case, there is also a second reason: I cannot ask for family-assisted suicide because it is not legally protected—a loved one who killed me might well be charged with murder. I could not ask my family to subject themselves to such a risk. Moreover, unlike physician-assisted suicide, we would not want to legalize family-assisted suicide. The lives of families are just too complex and too often laced with strong negative emotion—guilt, resentment, hatred, anger, desire for revenge. Family members also often have multiple motives stemming from deeply conflicting interests. As a result, there would be just too many cases in which family-assisted suicide would be indistinguishable from murder.[9]

Finally, family members may also fail. They also may lack know-how or bungle the job. Caught in the compelling emotions of grief and/or guilt, they may be unable to end a life that should be ended.

All this notwithstanding, family-assisted suicide may be the right choice, especially if physician-assisted suicide is unavailable. But should it be unavailable?

(3) Physician-assisted suicide: My doctor should kill me

There are, then, important difficulties with both unassisted suicide and family-assisted suicide. These difficulties are arguments for physician-assisted suicide and euthanasia. If my death comes too late, a physician is often the best candidate to kill me . . . or at the very least, to help me kill myself.

Perhaps the main argument for physician-assisted suicide grows out of the physician's extensive knowledge of disease and of dying. If it is a medical condition that leads me to contemplate ending my life, a key question for determining *when* or even *whether* I should end my life is: What is the prognosis? To what extent can my illness be treated or at least alleviated? How long do I have to live with my condition? How much worse will it get and how soon? What will life with that condition be like for me and my family? Few besides physicians possess all this critical information. I will be more likely to reach the right decision at the right time if a trusted physician is in on my plans to end my life.

A related point is physicians' knowledge of and access to drugs. Few of us know what drugs to take and in what amounts without the advice of a physician. Often, only a physician will know what to do to ensure that I do not vomit up the "suicide pill" or what to do if it fails. Physicians also have a monopoly on access to drugs. If my physician were more closely involved in the process, I could be more certain—and thus reassured—that my death will be peaceful and dignified, a death that permits reaffirmation of my connections with family and close friends.

A second argument for physician-assisted suicide grows out of physicians' greater experience with death and dying. Physicians know what to expect; those of us outside the health professions often do not. Granted, few physicians nowadays will know *me* and *my* family. For this reason, physicians should seldom make unilateral decisions about assisted suicide. Still, most physician could provide a rich source of information about death and about strategies to minimize the trauma, suffering, and agony of a death, both for the dying person and for the family.

Thirdly, physician-assisted suicide does not carry the same social stigma that unassisted suicide carries and physicians are not exposed to the legal risks involved in family-assisted suicide. Although many physicians are unwilling to take *any* risks to help someone end her life, there is really very little legal risk in physician-assisted suicide, especially if the family is in agreement. Physicians are also not morally censored the way family members would be for ending a life.

Finally, physicians ought not to abandon their patients, certainly not at the moment of death. Much has been made of the possibility that Americans would lose their trust in physicians if they knew that physicians sometimes kill. But many of us would trust our physicians *more* if we knew that we could count on them when death is needed or required (Quill and Cassell, 1995).

We have come, then, by a very round-about route to another argument for physician-assisted suicide. Often it is simply better— safer, more secure, more peaceful, less emotionally damaging for others—than unassisted suicide or family-assisted suicide. If physicians refuse to assist or are not permitted to do so, families and seriously ill people will be forced back on their own resources. And many deaths will be much worse than they need to be. When death comes too late, a physician will often be the best candidate to kill me.

And yet, physician-assisted suicide is not always the answer, either. Many physicians take themselves to be sworn to preserve human life in all its forms. Also, many people want doctors who are sworn not to kill, for fear that physicians might start making presumptuous, single-handed decisions about when death comes too late. Moreover, in a time when most people lack a significant personal relationship with their physicians, physician-assisted suicide is often a death that is remote, isolated, disconnected from the relationships that gave meaning to life. It is not always the best death. At times, then, family-assisted suicide and unassisted suicide remain the best answers.

CONCLUSION

We have a long cultural tradition of attempts to deal with the problems of death that comes too soon. Modern medicine, with its dramatic high-tech rescue attempts in the emergency room and the intensive care unit, is our society's attempt to prevent death from coming too soon. On a more personal level, we are bombarded with advice about ways to avoid a death that would be too soon—sooner than we wished, before we were ready for it.

We have much less cultural wisdom about the problems of a death that comes too late. It is almost as if we had spent all our cultural resources trying to avoid deaths that come too soon, only to find that we then had no resources left to help us when death comes too late.

Deaths that come too soon usually raise no difficult moral problems, however difficult they may be in other ways. Such deaths normally occur despite our best attempts to prevent them. "There's nothing more we can do," we say to the dying person, her family, and ourselves. And there is ethical solace in this, despite the tragedy of the death itself. We admit our failure. But our failure is not a moral failure—we did what we could.

Deaths that come too late are ethically much more troubling. They call on us to assume responsibility—to make difficult decisions and to do difficult things. We can try to hide from this responsibility by claiming that we should always try to prolong life, no matter what. Or by not deciding anything. But we know that not to decide is to decide. And it is very often just not clear what we should do. The weight of life-or-death decision pushes down upon us.

The recognition that the lives of members of families are intertwined makes the moral problems of a death that comes too late even more difficult. For they deprive us of our easiest and most comfortable answers—"it's up to the individual," "whatever the patient wants." But we do know that measures to improve or lengthen one life often compromise the quality of the lives of those to whom that person is connected.

So, we are morally troubled by deaths that come too late. We don't know what to do. Beyond that, the whole idea is unfamiliar to us. But in other societies—primarily technologically primitive and especially nomadic societies—almost everyone knew that death could come too late. People in those cultures knew that if they managed to live long enough, death would come too late and they would have to do something about it. They were prepared by their cultural traditions to find meaning in death and to do what needed to be done.

We have largely lost those traditions. Perhaps we have supposed that our wealth and technological sophistication have purchased exemption for us from any need to worry about living too long, from any need to live less than every minute we enjoy living. For a while it looked that way. But we must now face the fact: deaths that come too late are only the other side of our miraculous life-prolonging modern medicine.

We have so far avoided looking at this dark side of our medical triumphs. Our modern medicine saves many lives and enables us to live longer. That is wonderful, indeed. But it thereby also enables more of us to survive longer than we are able to care for ourselves, longer than we know what to do with ourselves, longer than we even *are* ourselves. Moreover, if further medical advances wipe out many of today's "killer diseases"—cancers, AIDS, heart attacks, etc.—then most of us will one day find that death is coming too late. And there will be a very common duty to die.

Our political system and health care reform (in the USA) are also moving in a direction that will put many more of us in the position of having a duty to die. Measures designed to control costs (for the government, and for employers who pay for retirement benefits and health insurance) often switch the burdens of care onto families. We are dismantling our welfare system and attempting to shift the costs of long-term health care onto families. One important consequence of these measures is that more of us will one day find ourselves a burden to our families and loved ones.[10]

Finally, we ourselves make choices that increase the odds that death will come too late. Patient autonomy gives us the right to make choices about our own medical treatment. We use that right to opt again and again for life-prolonging treatment—even when we have chronic illnesses, when we are debilitated, and as we begin to die. Despite this autonomy, we may feel we really have no choice, perhaps because we are unable to find meaning in death or to bring our lives to a meaningful close. But if we repeatedly opt for life-prolonging treatment, we thereby also increase the chances that death will come too late. This is the cost of patient autonomy, combined with powerful life-prolonging medical technology and inability to give meaning to death or even to accept it.

Death is very difficult for us. I have tried here to speak about it in plain language; I have used hard words and harsh tones to try to make us attend to troubling realities. We may question the arguments and conclusions of this paper. We should do so. But this questioning must not be fueled by denial or lead to evasion. For one thing seems very clear: we had better start learning how to deal with the problems of a death that comes too late. Some day, many of us will find that we should be dead or that one of our loved ones should be dead. What should we do then? We had better prepare ourselves—mentally, morally, culturally, spiritually, and socially. For many of us, if we are to die at the right time, it will be up to us.

ACKNOWLEDGMENTS

I get by with a little help from my friends. I wish to thank Hilde and Jim Nelson, Mary English, Tom Townsend, and Hugh LaFollette for helpful comments on earlier versions of this paper. And more: these friends have been my companions and guides throughout my attempt to think through the meaning of love and family in our lives.

NOTES

1. A note about language: I will be using "responsibility," "obligation," and "duty" interchangeably, despite significant differences in meaning. I generally use the word "duty" because it strikes me as a hard word for what can be a hard reality. (It also echoes Richard Lamm's famous statement that old people have a duty to die and get out of the way to give the next generation a chance.") Similarly, I use "kill" despite its connotations of destruction because I think we should not attempt to soften what we are doing. War and capital punishment have already taught us too much about how to talk in sweet and attractive ways about what we do. So I have resisted talking about "bringing my life to a close" and similar expressions. I have tried to use the plain, hard words.

2. There are many articles on this topic. Perhaps the classic article is Rachels (1975). It has been widely reprinted. A good collection of articles can be found in the *Journal of Medicine*

and Philosophy (June 1993), which was devoted to the topic, "Legal Euthanasia: Ethical Issues in an Era of Legalized Aid in Dying." Recent anthologies include Beauchamp (1996) and Moreno (1995).

3. A few states in the United States—currently (January 1996) New York, Missouri, Delaware, and Michigan—do require that family members be able to supply "clear and convincing evidence" that withdrawal of treatment is what their loved one would have wanted. This can be hard to prove. So it is especially important for those who live in these states to put their wishes about the kind of treatment they would want (if they become unable to decide for themselves) in writing. For information about the laws that apply in your state, write to Choice in Dying, 200 Varick Street, New York, NY 10014, or call them at 212-366-5540.

4. I believe we may also have a duty to ourselves to die, or a duty to the environment or a duty to the next generation to die. But I think for most of us, the strongest duty to die comes from our connections to family and loved ones, and this is the only source of a duty to die that I will consider here.

5. Most bioethicists advocate a "patient-centered ethics"—an ethics which claims only the patient's interests should be considered in making medical treatment decisions. Most health care professionals have been trained to accept this ethic and to see themselves as patient advocates. I have argued elsewhere that a patient-centered ethic is deeply mistaken. See Hardwig (1989) and Hardwig (1993).

6. I am considering only mentally competent adults. I do not think those who have never been competent—young children and those with severe retardation—can have moral duties. I do not know whether formerly competent people—e.g., those who have become severely demented—can still have moral duties. But if they cannot, I think some of us may face a duty to die even sooner—before we lose our moral agency.

7. A good account of the burdens of caregiving can be found in Brody (1990). To a large extent, care of the elderly is a women's issue. Most people who live to be 75 or older are women. But care for the elderly is almost always provided by women, as well—even when the person who needs care is the husband's parent.

8. Ultimately, in cases of deep and unresolvable disagreement between yourself and your loved ones, you may have to act on your own conception of your duty and your own conception of the burdens on them. But that is a fall-back position to resort to when the better, more relational ways of arriving at a belief in a duty to die fail or are unavailable.

9. Although this is true, we also need to rethink our reactions to the motives of the family. Because lives are intertwined, if someone "wants dad to be dead" and is relieved when he dies, this does not necessarily mean that she did not genuinely love him. Or that she is greedy, selfish, or self-centered. Her relief may stem from awareness of his suffering. It could also grow out of recognition of the sad fact that his life was destroying the lives of other family members whom she also loved.

10. Perhaps a more generous political system and a more equitable health care system could counteract the trend toward a more and more common duty to die. For now, at least, we could pay for the care of those who would otherwise be a burden on their families. If we were pre-

pared to do so, far fewer would face a duty to die. But we (in the US, at least) are not prepared to pay. Moreover, as medical advances enable more people to live longer (though also in various states of disability), it may be that the costs would overwhelm any society. Even if we could afford it, we should not continue to try to buy our way out of the problems of deaths that come too late. We would be foolish to devote all our resources to creating a society dedicated solely to helping all of us live just as long as we want.

REFERENCES

Beauchamp, T. L., ed. *Intending Death: The Ethics of Assisted Suicide and Euthanasia.* Englewood Cliffs, NJ: Prentice-Hall, 1996.

Brody, Elaine M. *Women in the Middle: Their Parent-Care Years.* New York: Springer, 1990.

Covinsky, Kenneth E., Goldman, Less, et al. "The Impact of a Serious Illness on Patients' Families." *Journal of the American Medical Association* 272 (1994), 1839–44.

Hardwig, John. "What About the Family?" *Hastings Center Report* 20 (March/April 1989): 5–10.

——."The Problem of Proxies with Interests of Their Own: Toward a Better Theory of Proxy Decisions." *Journal of Clinical Ethics* 4 (Spring 1993): 20–27.

Moreno, Jonathan, ed. *Arguing Euthanasia.* New York: Simon & Schuster, 1995.

Quill, Timothy E., and Cassell, Christine K. "Nonabandonment: A Central Obligation for Physicians," *Annals of Internal Medicine* 122 (1995): 368–74.

Rachels, James, "Active and Passive Euthanasia" *New England Journal of Medicine* 292 (1975): 78–80.

Smith, V. P. [pen name of Val Prendergrast]. "At Home with Alzheimer's," *Knoxville Metro Pulse*, 5, no.30 (1995): 7, 27.

Autobiography, Biography, and Narrative Ethics

There is, it seems to me, a preoccupation with autobiography in narrative bioethics. We need to overcome this preoccupation; autobiographies are both epistemically and morally suspect. Autobiographies remain important, of course, but biographies are also of critical importance, both for the theory of bioethics and for clinical practice. I take my concerns about autobiographies and an ethics based on them to be a concern *within* narrative ethics, not either an attack on it or a defense of it.

Before I begin, a word about how I will be using "narrative ethics." I do not include casuistry (*à la* Jonsen) within my purview.[1] Nor am I considering a view like Nussbaum's that reading literature is good for your character.[2] As will be clear from the examples I use, I am thinking primarily of the use of patients' stories of their lives and their illnesses. However, most of my reflections are general enough to apply to virtually any autobiographical account, and thus to narrative ethics beyond the field of bioethics.

The epistemic and moral weaknesses of autobiography are obvious and commonly recognized. I can claim no special insight here. In fact, once they stop to think about it, I expect most readers will have the sense that they were already aware of these problems.

One interesting question, then, is why narrative bioethics has not already recognized them. I cannot explore this issue in any depth. But I suggest that the causes may lie in our heritage of Cartesianism, together with a patient-centered bioethics. Failure to recognize the *epistemic* difficulties with autobiography seems to me to stem primarily from the ghosts of Cartesianism that continue to haunt us despite all our denials and attempts at exorcism. Blindness to the *moral* weaknesses of autobiography is, I believe, rooted in the much too simple patient-centered ethics that was traditional in medicine and has been taken over uncritically by contemporary bioethics. In its contemporary guise, a patient-centered ethics takes the form of an ethics centered in patient autonomy. Although Cartesianism and patient autonomy are largely separate traditions, they support each other in creating a focus on autobiography in bioethics.

The Epistemology of Autobiography

We are, often without even noticing it, still under the spell of two related Cartesian legacies: (1) Motives, interests, beliefs, desires, and attitudes are primarily mental states; action or behavior is, at most, an effect of these mental states. (2) Mental states exist in a consciousness, and since each of us is aware of our own consciousness, each of us knows her own beliefs, values, feelings, and so on. For convenience, I will call these twin Cartesian legacies the view that we are transparent to ourselves.

This Cartesian notion of self-transparency may seem doubly irrelevant to bioethics. In the first place, we deny that we accept any such pre-Freudian, pre-Hegelian (pre-Socratic?) notions. And, on some level, we do reject them. But they are deeply embedded in our common sense and our culture. Consequently, unless we are constantly vigilant, we find ourselves falling victim to this heritage despite ourselves. Secondly, Cartesian self-transparency may also seem remote from narrative bioethics because we deal in ethics, not epistemology. But ethics is not independent of epistemology. As I shall try to indicate, this tradition is neither remote nor irrelevant.

Within these Cartesian premises, the problem of knowledge is the problem of knowing whether there is a correspondence between our own consciousness and something outside it. Thus each of us knows her own mind, but there is a major problem of knowing other minds. We have direct access to our own consciousness but none to someone else's, and inferences from behavior—including verbal behavior—to mental states are always precarious. Each of us is thus in a position of unique epistemic authority with respect to our own minds—your knowledge of my beliefs, desires, motives, intentions can never be better than mine. Indeed, your knowledge (if any) is derivative from mine, depending as it does on my reports about my mental states.

Within narrative bioethics, this Cartesian legacy yields a nearly exclusive fascination with autobiography. Autobiographies are authoritative. The stories we are concerned with, the stories that are to figure in narrative ethics are *the patient*'s stories—as told by the patient, of course. If there is no problem with knowing our own minds, but major obstacles to knowing the minds of others, then autobiographies are the stories we need, the stories to rely on in narrative ethics.

Were we not under the Cartesian spell, we would immediately recognize this as palpably naïve. The authoritative account of someone's life is her own—her autobiography? Of course not! In our everyday lives and dealings with each other, nobody would take a first-person account as the definitive or even the most reliable word on the subject. "I am the only one at work who understands the business." Hmm. "I was just trying to help her get control of her life." I wonder. "My ex-wife. . . ."—*whatever* follows that expression is deeply suspect. Would anyone be fool enough to take a former President's autobiography as the definitive account of what he was doing while he was President?

We may think that President Nixon's account of his White House years is riddled with lies. But lies are only one problem and they arise only at the final stage, the stage at which I tell my story for others. But autobiography plays an earlier and more basic role, too—I tell the story of my life *for myself*. The narrative we tell about ourselves is part of living a life that is *a life*, with unity and coherence, rather than just a bunch of experiences that happened to the same person.

The fact that we tell—and perhaps must tell—ourselves stories about our lives introduces an important ambiguity into what we mean by autobiography. The story I tell myself about my life is not an autobiography to which you can ever have access—probably not even if we are intimate, certainly not if we are strangers. We all have secrets. So you must be content with the story I tell for public consumption. That will not normally be exactly the way I see my life. The autobiographies we can consider in bioethics are thus all "secondhand" autobiographies, stories retold for an external audience. They may contain lies and distortions; they will normally be crafted for their intended audience. We shall return to this point.

First, however, if we escape the spell of Cartesianism, we quickly see that even the stories we tell ourselves contain lies and distortions. Self-deception is an important feature of our lives and an important phenomenon for an evaluation of autobiographies. In fact, there are at least four different sets of epistemic problems with autobiographies: (1) ignorance; (2) innocent mistakes; (3) self-deception; and finally (4) lies. Let us briefly consider each of these.

Ignorance and innocent mistakes are the simplest of these problems, so let's start here. There are many things that we do not know about events in our lives. What I do not know cannot figure in my autobiography, however important it may be to my life. I do not know why my former wife finally decided to move to California with me, or why the philosophy department at Humboldt State voted not to renew my contract. Both are important turning points in any story of my life. Which story I choose to tell may well turn on my beliefs about why these pivotal decisions were made as they were.

Notice, too, that some of the things I do not know about my life I could not even find out . . . without relying on someone else (a biographer, perhaps). Someone else might be able to elicit a much more straightforward and truthful account of important events in my life. My former wife may, for example, tell others things about our relationship that she would never tell me. My autobiography is, then, epistemically limited, not only by my ignorance, but by information unavailable to me, though perhaps available to others.

These are failures to know *others* completely enough. But even more important is the fact that there is also much about ourselves that we do not know. We are not close to being transparent to ourselves. There is much about even our present state of mind that we do not know. This is true even on a very basic level. Many discussions of informed consent seem to be plagued by the assumption that the patient will know what treatment she wants if she is just informed about the pros and cons of the various options. But even outside of a medical context, it is often hard for me to know what I want. The problem here is not only one of envisioning what life would be like under various conditions. Nor am I playing on some fancy notion of what I *really* want. It's simply that I often have trouble knowing what I want right now.

Of course, telling the story of my life requires knowing much more about me than just my present state of consciousness. And as we move into less basic though equally critical elements of my account of myself, the likelihood of errors multiplies rapidly. I am quite capable of major mistakes about my beliefs and values. My own account of my intentions, my motives, my character, my personality are all extremely unreliable. The rage I feel is unnoticed, my desire for revenge unexperienced, and consequently my account of what I was up to is . . . not only fallible, not only faulty or flawed, but fundamentally wrong and wrongheaded. I used to divide the world into "settlers" and "explorers" and thought of myself as an explorer. My partner just hooted at that idea. And she was right.

Thus either desires, motives, beliefs, values, and attitudes are not mental states at all, or I can be mistaken about my own mental states. In addition, we have an "outside," as it were, not just an inside. We are normally known at least as much by what we do as by what we say about ourselves. And what I do is a public phenomenon, not uniquely or immediately accessible to me. I have direct access *at most* to what I intended to do, and if my desire for revenge can be unexperienced by me, I may not know even that. Indeed, on some epistemologies—notably Mead's—it is only through the responses of others that I come to have knowledge even of what I am saying (as opposed to merely thinking), and thinking is itself derivative from saying.[3]

So much for innocent mistakes. They are innocent and thus not very interesting, though they do raise interesting problems for a narrative ethics based on autobiography. Yet perhaps the most interesting thing to be said about innocent mistakes is that it is hard to find a really convincing example of one. *Why* did you not notice your rage? Everyone else did! And how *could* you have overlooked your desire for revenge? It colored virtually everything you did! You, an *explorer? You?*

The important mistakes in my autobiography may not be innocent. I have an important stake in which story I tell about my life. As a result, autobiographies are often—even standardly—riddled with self-deception. Self-deception is motivated, not innocent. If I am telling the story and the story is about me, I will normally want to leave the audience with a favorable impression about the central character. The first audience of my story is myself, and I desperately want to feel good about myself. The stories I tell myself are imbued with that mission.

Most of us do in fact manage to cast ourselves in a favorable light, at least to ourselves. (Even those who are habitually "down on themselves" usually feel that they are more honest with themselves or have higher moral standards than those who feel good about themselves.) Self-assessment and self-judgment are always epistemically suspect; consequently, autobiography is, in important respects, seldom the most trustworthy story of a life. In fact, one of the reasons I often do not even know what I want is because I have many wants that I don't want to admit to myself.

Let's move on now to stories told for others. I am also very much interested in what the broader, outside audience thinks of me. I would like to leave a good impression. I want almost everyone to be impressed with me and what I have done, everyone to think well of me, everyone to like me. The first thing this causes me to do is to tell my story in light of the ideas I have about the beliefs and values of the audience. I tell different stories for different audiences, and they may all be inaccurate, if only by reason of onesidedness.

Joanne Lynn argues that most seriously ill and dying patients are desperately trying to be "a good patient."[4] They very much want to do a good job of dying in the eyes of doctors, family, and friends—the audiences. After all, this is their last chance to do well, their last chance to leave a good impression, their only chance to die well. If Lynn is correct, the autobiographies of terminally ill people—including their statements about what kind of treatment they want—will usually be decisively shaped by this desire to meet the norms and expectations of different audiences. Viewed in this light, it may not be surprising that many patients tell one story to one doctor, another to another, yet a third to a nurse, and still other stories to various members of their families. If I detect different expectations, I will tell different stories.

Of course, a variety of stories *may* all be true. All stories of a life are incomplete (or they would take about as long to tell as to live). And it may be that different stories—different emphases perhaps—are appropriate for different audiences and different purposes. I know, for example, that you are a clinician and you are interested in a story focused on health and illness. So I may leave things completely out of my story that are much more important to me than my health. But my motivation in shaping my story to its audience is also normally not purely altruistic. I edit, shade, stretch, distort, and often even lie in an attempt to secure a more favorable response from my various audiences.

Now, lies and self-deception are intimately related. There are at least three important feedback loops between the stories I tell for various audiences and my self-knowledge. First, it is much easier for me to tell you a story that you will find convincing if I believe it myself. Consequently, I can easily fall victim to my attempts to impress or deceive you and end up believing the stories I have told for public consumption. Lying often ends in self-deception.

Second, my desire to leave a favorable impression on you is deeply confusing to me—it makes it harder for me to distinguish my own wants from your expectations or hopes of me. When a patient opts for more treatment for her cancer, how, then, can we assume that she knows what *she* wants, as opposed to wanting what she thinks we expect of her? Lynn thinks she may well not know what she wants. Of course, she may want most *whatever* will leave a favorable impression on the audience. But presumably our ethics of informed consent is not to reduce to an elaborate game in which patients are forced to try to guess what medical treatment we want them to choose.

Third, partly as a result of these first two feedback loops, there may well be limits to how long and how thoroughly I can tell a story for public consumption without becoming what I pretend to be. A very dramatic example is provided by police who work with undercover agents. The very lives of undercover narcotics agents, for example, depend on their ability to tell their cover stories convincingly. Police officers relate that an agent–any agent, anyone—can go underground for only about 6 months before she literally loses track of who she is.[5] She will, for example, no longer remember that she is a police officer or who her father is. And if we believe that the story we tell about ourselves is the basis of identity, we will be forced to conclude that an agent can only go underground for about 6 months before she *becomes* a different person.

So much for a brief overview of ignorance, mistakes, self-deception, and lies in autobiographies. There is one more reason for concern about the epistemic trustworthiness of autobiographical accounts: I am normally the central character in my autobiography. But if I see myself as the central character, won't my account tend to overplay the importance of my own role and contribution, and correspondingly to underrate the place and contribution of others? Thus, when I tell the story of the philosophy department at East Tennessee State University during my years as chair, it tends to place too much emphasis on what I did.

MULTIPLE AUTOBIOGRAPHIES

Autobiographies contain many epistemic weaknesses; they are all epistemically suspect. But even if they are often mistaken, isn't there something privileged about autobiographies? Right or wrong, honest or distorted, an autobiography is, after all, the way *I* see my life; it expresses the meaning my life has for me. And that is what is important for stories of illness and for medical treatment decisions.

But we have already seen that the autobiography I tell myself is not available to you. Should we even say that the story I tell *myself* is the way *I* see my life? "How could it fail to be the way I see my life? My conscious experiences are my conscious experiences, after all! The way I see myself and my life may be mistaken, but it *is* the way I see it!" But that is the voice of the Cartesian legacy again. If we recognize self-deception, doesn't "the story I tell myself" become systematically ambiguous? If my desire for revenge colors virtually everything I do but I deny this to myself, or if I see myself as an explorer but unfailingly choose the familiar and the secure . . . what are we to say?

I think we must say that I am telling myself at least *two* stories simultaneously, one in which the desire for revenge does not figure at all, but also another in which it looms large and is justified. But I am unaware of this second story, unaware of it despite the fact that I am telling it! Strange as this may seem, I think we *must* say that I am telling myself multiple stories, for my *action* (as opposed to my deceptive conscious awareness) is also story-driven. It, too, has narrative unity.

Now, if you take my conscious story that I do not seek revenge as the whole of my story or even the center of it, you will treat me inappropriately, and I will be disappointed, frustrated, or enraged by what you do. For the stories I *consciously* tell myself will be only one part of my own sense of my life. I can articulate for myself only some of the meaning my life has for me; some of that meaning I may be quite unaware of. Thus, dealing most sensitively and effectively with a self-deceived, inarticulate, or unreflective person—any of us to some extent—will involve attempting to ferret out *all* the stories she tells herself, including those she is not aware of.

The meaning my own life has for me is thus never completely captured in the stories I am aware of. Self-knowledge, on the account I am suggesting, would involve coming to acknowledge this multiplicity of autobiographies, learning to ferret out and articulate all of them, dealing with the discrepancies among them, and then ceasing to tell oneself the self-deceptive stories. Only with perfect self-knowledge would my autobiography be single, and only then would it accurately convey the complete sense or meaning my life has for me.

AUTOBIOGRAPHY AND THE CLINICAL ENCOUNTER

Exclusive reliance upon patient autobiographies would do more than place narrative ethics on a perilous epistemic foundation. It would weaken the practice of medicine, as well. Wherever accuracy is important, there are serious questions about whether we ought to attend exclusively—or even primarily—to autobiography. Consider, first, small things. Medical students are taught to double the amount of alcohol I say I consume and perhaps also the number of cigarettes I say I smoke. The veracity of the sexual history I give is suspect, as is the story I tell about what I eat or why I am seeking pain medication. Users of illegal substances often deny use. Child abuse, spouse abuse, and elder abuse invite cover stories.

Consider next the following examples: "He says that he hates his job and being on disability would be wonderful. But I know how depressed he is whenever he can't work and how horrible he feels about himself when he doesn't have a job." "He'll tell you that impotence is no big deal at his age, but it bothers him tremendously." "She says she's doing OK, but she stays drunk or high most of the time since her accident." "He says his memory is pretty good, but I'm afraid to leave him alone for even a few hours." "She says she still gets around pretty well, but there are many days when she can barely make it to the bathroom and back. She wants you to think she can take care of herself because she's terrified of going into a nursing home."

Moreover, because health, sickness, and medicine often touch on very intimate features of our lives, they evoke all kinds of very basic attitudes about what is appropriate to tell to whom and how the audience will evaluate me if I reveal this fact about myself. I have seen patients who are unable or unwilling to admit the amount of pain they are suffering for fear of being thought weak or unmanly. Bulimia is something many young women cannot talk about. The spectacle of my death may be too terrifying to mention. Or I may be too ashamed of my terror to mention that.

We have seen that the story a clinician or bioethicist receives is seldom the story the patient tells herself. It may well not be the story the patient would tell another audience. But even if a clinician could elicit the story I consciously tell myself, that would normally not fully capture the meaning my life and action have for me. For all these reasons, sensitive and appropriate treatment of me in the clinic or hospital depends—just as it does in other contexts—on a careful attempt to weave a coherent picture of me and my illness out of the various stories I tell, together with the stories others tell about me.

The import of these points runs deep. In light of the multiple stories I will usually be telling myself and others, how do you respect or honor my autonomy? How do you design a plan of medical treatment for me that will embody or promote the meaning my life has for me? Do you attend only to the story I tell you? If so, why am I so upset when you treat me like the explorer I take myself to be? Or must you also consider the stories I tell others and even try to gain access to the stories that inform my action but not my awareness of myself? If the latter, you must talk with my partner, not just me—she will readily tell you that I am certainly no explorer, however much I may see myself that way. Thus, even promoting patient autonomy must not rest solely on autobiography. If you would respect or promote my autonomy, you must attend to various *biographies* of me, not just to the story I consciously tell myself . . . or you.

Good clinicians must, then, be skilled biographers, not just faithful receptors of patient autobiographies.6 Part of the training of medical, nursing, and social work students must be—and already is—developing their skills as biographers. In this respect, the practice of medicine and nursing may well be far more sophisticated than our theories of narrative bioethics that are rooted in patient autobiographies.

THE MORAL EVALUATION OF AUTOBIOGRAPHIES

We have so far considered mainly the implications for me of treating me on the basis of my autobiography. Let us now turn to the implications *for others* of my autobiography. With this we move to a more straightforwardly *moral* evaluation of autobiography. We can begin by reflecting on the central role I assign myself in the story I tell about my life: *Shouldn't* I be the central character in the story of *my* life? Especially if it's the story of my life *as told by me!* Isn't there something pathetic or deeply unfortunate about those who do not play the central role even in their own autobiographies? Moreover, don't I have some fundamental right to tell the story of my life? Whose life is it, anyway?

But I am not the only character in my story. The story of my life cannot be simply the story of me, for there is no way to separate my life from the lives of those around me and especially those intimately connected with me. Any story of my life will have to include many other characters. Let's focus our reflections on the role of family and loved ones in my autobiography, since their lives are most closely intertwined with mine, and they are the ones most likely to be deeply affected by the role I assign them in the story I tell.

In contrast with autobiography, there is in many joint endeavors or communities no central character. Often, there is no central character in a neighborhood, an academic department, a business, a government agency, or a team. That's usually an important part of what makes them healthy. Certainly there is no central character in a healthy family.

Another part of what makes families healthy is that there is, in important respects, not one story for each family member, but only one story among them. The claim that there should be (in many significant respects) only one story in a family is not the claim that families should be monolithic entities, committed to one set of beliefs and values, with no tolerance for deviance. There can be difference, conflict, even basically different perspectives within one story. Rather, the point is that families (couples, friendships) in which too many different stories are told are typically characterized by lack of communication and understanding, and also by an absence of intimacy and sharing.

Who tells the story when lives are intertwined? It is a privilege and a power to have the right to tell the story. In other contexts, it is normally the privilege of the powerful—the dominant man—to tell the official story of "his" family and "his" family life. But in bioethics, we listen to the patient's story.

Reliance upon patients' autobiographies both reflects and reinforces a patient-centered bioethics. The patient-centered feature of bioethics seems entirely justified and even noble—it's just advocacy for the vulnerable. But in bioethics, as elsewhere, when we attend exclusively to one family member's story, we tend to ignore or discount the ramifications on the lives of the rest of the family.[7] They are only bit players of marginal importance in the story we are concerned with. Exclusive reliance upon autobiography thus systematically undervalues others and overlooks or discounts the importance of their interests.

There are at least two forms of oppression involved in reliance upon any one family member's story.

First, it silences the others. A focus on *the patient*'s autobiography silences all other members of her family. *Their* interests and *their* autobiographies do not count. And the family *is* in fact all too effectively silenced by our bioethics and in our health care system. Decisions are made every day that promote the patient's interests at truly staggering costs to the lives of other members of the patient's family. These decisions are routinely made as if families were no more than patient support systems or as if the interests of other members of the family were somehow morally irrelevant. We do not even ask whether it is morally legitimate to impose these burdens on the patient's family—in fact, a patient-centered ethics implicitly *requires* that we not consider the interests of the family. Because our ethics has so thoroughly silenced families, we can congratulate ourselves on an ethics that places the patient's interests over all others and on having faithfully served the patient's interests.

But it is wrong to consider only the well-being of one member of a family when the lives of the others will also be dramatically affected. To do so is tacitly to reduce all other family members to means to the well-being of the one family member who is ill. Because this is wrong, it is also wrong to listen exclusively to the patient's story. Doing so always runs the risk of inappropriately discounting the interests of the rest of the family.

All this is true of the autobiographies we tell when we are at our best. Even at our best, most of us assign ourselves the central role in our stories. Most of us are inclined to weigh benefits and burdens to ourselves more heavily than those to others. We all tend to be self-centered. But if illness makes most people more self-absorbed, self-centered, or inconsiderate, more regressed into a primitive or immature self, then the autobiographies of the seriously or chronically ill will be especially likely to shortchange the interests of others. And all of this is further reinforced by an audience of health care professionals and bioethicists who are most interested in the health-related aspects and outcomes of the story and who are all professionally committed to weighing in on the side of the sick. For these reasons, we should be especially wary of relying on a sick person's story.

But even when the interests of others are not inappropriately discounted in the story, it is still a form of oppression for any one person to tell the official story of a group—family, clan, business, team, government, or ethics consult. It is not, for example, morally sufficient if I paternalistically take the interests of the rest of my family into consideration, not even if I am scrupulously fair in doing so.

They must be allowed to speak for themselves—to define their own interests, to say how they see our present situation. Allowing others also to tell their version of the story is part of what is involved in respecting them as persons. Thus there is a basic moral criticism of exclusive attention to anyone's autobiography . . . with the possible exception of those who are all alone, with no family, friends, or loved ones.

The second way in which people can be oppressed by an autobiography is that they can be forced to live in someone else's story. This form of oppression grows out of the fact that we are not only passive tellers of our stories, but also active agents who are living our lives. We all attempt to live out a script. In order to continue to live our present script, we must often try to fit recalcitrant reality into our stories. One option for fitting reality into a story is, as we have seen, deception and self-deception. But as actors, we have a second option for fitting reality into our scripts. We can actively shape reality to fit the story we are telling. This is not in itself remarkable, uncommon, or morally troublesome; it is an essential feature of action, an inescapable part of forging a life.

But it can easily slide into a form of oppression: We attempt to force others to live as characters in our stories. Take the example—perhaps the caricature—of the traditional husband who "takes care of the little woman." If I am living out that style of masculinity, then I *must* see my wife as "the little woman"—as needing help, perhaps even as fundamentally incapable of taking care of herself. Otherwise the story I am attempting to live out will lapse into incoherence, and a large part of my life becomes meaningless. I may, as a result, take steps to make reality conform to this perception. I take steps—normally without full awareness of what I am doing—that tend to incapacitate my wife in order that I may be the man who takes care of her. This sometimes takes truly horrific forms. Equally horrific, to mention just one more example, are attempts to create my sons in my own image, to make them "chips off the old block."

(Distance normally insulates outsiders to some extent; they are somewhat more immune than family members to this sort of oppression. But outsiders, too, can be forced to live in the stories of others. In fact, the frustration physicians and nurses feel over providing futile treatment can be a result of the professional debasement that can result when health care professionals are forced to play an assigned role in the patient's or family's preferred story.)

To the extent that I am successful in forcing, manipulating, pressuring, or badgering others to live as characters in my story, I deprive them of the opportunity to author their own stories. There is a fundamental loss of freedom and autonomy in this. It is, at bottom, to deprive the other of the opportunity to live her own life. Although illness can help to free other members of my family from this form of tyranny, it can also serve to strengthen my hand in making them serve my story. Ideally, of course, we should be creating a story *together.*

To summarize, the moral challenge to a narrative ethics based on patient autobiography is that it harbors two forms of oppression. First, others are silenced and often slighted if only my story about our life together is attended to. It is wrong to slight the interests of others; it is wrong to silence others even if they are not slighted as a result. Secondly, I easily wrong others by attempting to mold them to fit into my story. Others aid and abet both forms of oppression if they attend exclusively or even primarily to the story I tell about my life and the place others have in it. For these two reasons, a narrative bioethics based primarily on patient autobiography is morally as well as epistemologically flawed.

THE ALTERNATIVE

What is the alternative to a preoccupation with autobiographies in narrative ethics? I have already hinted at it. The alternative is to acknowledge that an autobiography is only *one* account of a life, a deeply fallible and often unreliable account at that. Moreover, all of us live in and tell many autobiographies. Consequently, insofar as narrative bioethics requires an accurate account of a life or an illness, we need to piece together the narrative by attending to many stories told by many tellers. Acknowledging this would involve coming to see that the patient's *husband* has a perfectly valid "take" on her wishes and values, on what her life has been all about, on "what she is up to" (including what she is up to in telling her story the way she does).

Of course, the point here is not that we are transparent to *others* but not to ourselves. There are limits to others' knowledge of me, too. Other narrators also have agendas; their stories about me also contain mistakes. Their stories are also motivated, shaped for an intended audience, designed to impress us with the narrator, and so on.

This is true even for those of us famous or distinguished enough to have professional—"detached," "objective"—biographers. It is even more true of biographers with whom we have had extended interaction. My physician, in telling the story of my case, is also inevitably telling a story about how she practices medicine and even about who she is. And the biographers who have most at stake in telling our stories one way rather than another are our more common "intimate biographers"—lovers, close friends, and family members. Their self-images and even their lives may turn dramatically on the way they tell the story about us.

There is, then, no detached observer—value-free, motiveless, with no intentions, no plans, no agenda— to tell the authoritative story.[8] There is no authoritative story. Because there is no "view from nowhere," the alternative to autobiography in narrative ethics cannot be simply a return to the physician's privilege to tell the story of the case. Rather, we must recognize that the physician—or bioethicist—tells the story of patients in the way she does because of the limits of her own self-knowledge and the agendas she brings to bear. The person cannot be left out of the story she tells; the person cannot really even be left out of the factual or scientific observations she makes about the case.

This more complex view of narrative and narrative ethics requires a new discipline of us. There may well still be a point to the traditional discipline of trying to achieve and speak from a detached, value-free standpoint. Often we should try to put ourselves out of play in telling stories about others, or even about ourselves. But recognizing that we all inevitably fail to achieve an objective, detached, unmotivated account either of ourselves or of others, we need also to learn another, rather different discipline—that of coming to recognize our own motivations, biases, agendas, and then of stating them quite explicitly. This kind of self-knowledge is required of a narrator—and thus of a health care professional—if her account is to be maximally reliable and morally trustworthy.

If someone has the requisites that enable her to offer an epistemically reliable and morally trustworthy autobiography, it will be because she has long participated in a complex, multiperson process, listening to many different accounts of her dreams, fears, plans, actions, activities, and past. She knows herself because she continually tries out various versions of her story—biographies are well as autobiographies—on many audiences to check the reliability of her own view against their responses to what she is saying about her life.[9]

Autobiographies that are both epistemically and morally reliable are thus derivative from biographies: It is only through having attended to many stories about me—including the stories others tell in response to my earlier autobiographies—that I can finally give a trustworthy account of my own life. Still, self-knowledge is never complete. No one's autobiography should ever be taken as the definitive account of her life. And none of us can completely avoid deeply troubling and pervasive forms of oppression that often pass unnoticed in the stories we tell.

In light of all this, we might venture a fundamental reinterpretation of autonomy, including patient autonomy. The autonomous person is not an island or some transparent self who has immediate knowledge of what goes on inside herself and who clings to that in the face of everything anyone else may say. No, an autonomous person develops an autobiography in community—in this complex, multiperson encounter seeking the truth about her and her life with others. On this alternative view, only those who have participated in such a process can become autonomous. For it is only through hearing many stories about ourselves that we can know ourselves, what our life has been . . . or even what it means to us.

The art of weighing these many different and often conflicting stories, and of weaving them together into a reasonably coherent though multivocal account, is the art of the biographer. As bioethicists and clinicians we must, then, become biographers, not simply faithful recorders of autobiographies. Listening to multiple sources is epistemically more reliable than exclusive reliance upon any one source. Attending to many voices is almost always morally preferable to listening to only one. Dialogue is better than monologue.

Acknowledgments

I wish to thank Hugh LaFollette, Stuart Finder, and Hilde Nelson for helpful comments on earlier versions of this paper.

Notes

1. Albert Jonsen, and Stephen Toulmin. *The Abuse of Casuistry: A History of Moral Reasoning.* Berkeley: University of California Press, 1988.

2. Martha Nussbaum. Poetic Justice: *The Literary Imagination and Public Life.* Boston: Beacon, 1995.

3. George Herbert Mead. *Mind, Self, and Society*. Chicago: U of Chicago P, 1962.

4. Joanne Lynn. "End of Life Decision Making in Seriously Ill Patients." Presented at "Deciding How We Die: The Use and Limits of Advance Directives," Roanoke, VA, 15 Sept. 1995, conference sponsored by Carilion Health Systems.

5. I owe this point to Edwin J. Delattre, in conversation.

6. I owe this point to William Donnally, in conversation.

7. For an argument that a patient-centered ethic should be replaced by a family-centered ethic, see John Hardwig. "What about the Family?" *Hastings Center Report* 20.2 (1990): 3–10; Hilde L. Nelson, and James L. Nelson. *The Patient in the Family*. New York: Routledge, 1995.

8. It should be obvious by now—if not long before—that this paper is deeply indebted to feminist epistemology. See, for example, Sandra Harding. *Whose Science? Whose Knowledge? Thinking From Women's Lives*. Ithaca, NY: Cornell U P, 1991.

9. I have argued that dialogue is necessary for self-knowledge and thus for moral rationality in a very early article: John Hardwig. "The Achievement of Moral Rationality," *Philosophy & Rhetoric* 6 (1973): 171–85.

Is There a Duty to Die?

When Richard Lamm made the statement that old people have a duty to die, it was generally shouted down or ridiculed. The whole idea is just too preposterous to entertain. Or too threatening. In fact, a fairly common argument against legalizing physician-assisted suicide is that if it were legal, some people might somehow get the idea that they have a duty to die. These people could only be the victims of twisted moral reasoning or vicious social pressure. It goes without saying that there is no duty to die.

But for me the question is real and very important. I feel strongly that I may very well some day have a duty to die. I do not believe that I am idiosyncratic, morbid, mentally ill, or morally perverse in thinking this. I think many of us will eventually face precisely this duty. But I am first of all concerned with my own duty. I write partly to clarify my own convictions and to prepare myself. Ending my life might be a very difficult thing for me to do.

This notion of a duty to die raises all sorts of interesting theoretical and metaethical questions. I intend to try to avoid most of them because I hope my argument will be persuasive to those holding a wide variety of ethical views. Also, although the claim that there is a duty to die would ultimately require theoretical underpinning, the discussion needs to begin on the normative level. As is appropriate to my attempt to steer clear of theoretical commitments, I will use "duty," "obligation," and "responsibility" interchangeably, in a pretheoretical or preanalytic sense.[1]

CIRCUMSTANCES AND A DUTY TO DIE

Do many of us really believe that no one ever has a duty to die? I suspect not. I think most of us probably believe that there is such a duty, but it is very uncommon. Consider Captain Oates, a member of Admiral Scott's expedition to the South Pole. Oates became too ill to continue. If the rest of the team stayed with him, they would all perish. After this had become clear, Oates left his tent one night, walked out into a raging blizzard, and was never seen again.[2] That may have been a heroic thing to do, but we might be able to agree that it was also no more than his duty. It would have been wrong for him to urge—or even to allow—the rest to stay and care for him.

This is a very unusual circumstance—a "lifeboat case"—and lifeboat cases make for bad ethics. But I expect that most of us would also agree that there have been cultures in which what we would call a duty to die has been fairly common. These are relatively poor, technologically simple, and especially nomadic cultures. In such societies, everyone knows that if you manage to live long enough, you will eventually become old and debilitated. Then you will need to take steps to end your life. The old people in these societies regularly did precisely that. Their cultures prepared and supported them in doing so.

Those cultures could be dismissed as irrelevant to contemporary bioethics; their circumstances are so different from ours. But if that is our response, it is instructive. It suggests that we assume a duty to die is irrelevant to us because our wealth and technological sophistication have purchased exemption for us . . . except under very unusual circumstances like Captain Oates's.

But have wealth and technology really exempted us? Or are they, on the contrary, about to make a duty to die common again? We like to think of modern medicine as all triumph with no dark side. Our medicine saves many lives and enables most of us to live longer. That is wonderful, indeed. We are all glad to have access to this medicine. But our medicine also delivers most of us over to chronic illnesses and it enables many of us to survive longer than we can take care of ourselves, longer than we know what to do with ourselves, longer than we even are ourselves.

The costs—and these are not merely monetary—of prolonging our lives when we are no longer able to care for ourselves are often staggering. If further medical advances wipe out many of today's "killer diseases"—cancers, heart attacks, strokes, ALS, AIDS, and the rest—then one day most of us will survive long enough to become demented or debilitated. These developments could generate a fairly widespread duty to die. A fairly common duty to die might turn out to be only the dark side of our life-prolonging medicine and the uses we choose to make of it.

Let me be clear. I certainly believe that there is a duty to refuse life-prolonging medical treatment and also a duty to complete advance directives refusing life-prolonging treatment. But a duty to die can go well beyond that. There can be a duty to die before one's illnesses would cause death, even if treated only with palliative measures. In fact, there may be a fairly common responsibility to end one's life in the absence of any terminal illness at all. Finally, there can be a duty to die when one would prefer to live. Granted, many of the conditions that can generate a duty to die also seriously undermine the quality of life. Some prefer not to live under such conditions. But even those who want to live can face a duty to die. These will clearly be the most controversial and troubling cases; I will, accordingly, focus my reflections on them.

The Individualistic Fantasy

Because a duty to die seems such a real possibility to me, I wonder why contemporary bioethics has dismissed it without serious consideration. I believe that most bioethics still shares in one of our deeply embedded American dreams: the individualistic fantasy. This fantasy leads us to imagine that lives are separate and unconnected, or that they could be so if we chose. If lives were unconnected, things that happened in my life would not or need not affect others. And if others were not (much) affected by my life, I would have no duty to consider the impact of my decisions on others. I would then be free morally to live my life however I please, choosing whatever life and death I prefer for myself. The way I live would be nobody's business but my own. I certainly would have no duty to die if I preferred to live.

Within a health care context, the individualistic fantasy leads us to assume that the patient is the only one affected by decisions about her medical treatment. If only the patient were affected, the relevant questions when making treatment decisions would be precisely those we ask: What will benefit the patient? Who can best decide that? The pivotal issue would always be simply whether the patient wants to live like this and whether she would consider herself better off dead.[3] "Whose life is it, anyway?" we ask rhetorically.

But this is morally obtuse. We are not a race of hermits. Illness and death do not come only to those who are all alone. Nor is it much better to think in terms of the bald dichotomy between "the interests of the patient" and "the interests of society" (or a third-party payer), as if we were isolated individuals connected only to "society" in the abstract or to the other, faceless members of our health maintenance organization.

Most of us are affiliated with particular others and most deeply, with family and loved ones. Families and loved ones are bound together by ties of care and affection, by legal relations and obligations, by inhabiting shared spaces and living units, by interlocking finances and economic prospects, by common projects and also commitments to support the different life projects of other family members, by shared histories, by ties of loyalty. This life together of family and loved ones is what defines and sustains us; it is what gives meaning to most of our lives. We would not have it any other way. We would not want to be all alone, especially when we are seriously ill, as we age, and when we are dying.

But the fact of deeply interwoven lives debars us from making exclusively self-regarding decisions, as the decisions of one member of a family may dramatically affect the lives of all the rest. The impact of my decisions upon my family and loved ones is the source of many of my strongest obligations and also the most plausible and likeliest basis of a duty to die. "Society," after all, is only very marginally affected by how I live, or by whether I live or die.

A Burden to My Loved Ones

Many older people report that their one remaining goal in life is not to be a burden to their loved ones. Young people feel this, too: When I ask my undergraduate students to think about whether their death could come too late, one of their very first responses always is, "Yes, when I become a burden to my family or loved ones." Tragically, there are situations in which my loved ones would be much better off—all things considered, the loss of a loved one notwithstanding—if I were dead.

The lives of our loved ones can be seriously compromised by caring for us. The burdens of providing care or even just supervision 24 hours a day, 7 days a week are often overwhelming.[4] When this kind of caregiving goes on for years, it leaves the caregiver exhausted, with no time for herself or life of her own. Ultimately, even her health is often destroyed. But it can also be emotionally devastating simply to live with a spouse who is increasingly distant, uncommunicative, unresponsive, foreign, and unreachable. Other family members' needs often go unmet as the caring capacity of the family is exceeded. Social life and friendships evaporate, as there is no opportunity to go out to see friends and the home is no longer a place suitable for having friends in.

We must also acknowledge that the lives of our loved ones can be devastated just by having to pay for health care for us. One part of the recent SUPPORT study documented the financial aspects of caring for a dying member of a family. Only those who had illnesses severe enough to give them less than a 50 percent chance to live 6 more months were included in this study. When these patients survived their initial hospitalization and were discharged about one-third required considerable caregiving from their families; in 20 percent of cases a family member had to quit work or make some other major lifestyle change; almost one-third of these families lost all of their savings; and just under 30 percent lost a major source of income.[5]

If talking about money sounds venal or trivial, remember that much more than money is normally at stake here. When someone has to quit work, she may well lose her career. Savings decimated late in life cannot be recouped in the few remaining years of employability, so the loss compromises the quality of the rest of the caregiver's life. For a young person, the chance to go to college may be lost to the attempt to pay debts due to an illness in the family, and this decisively shapes an entire life.

A serious illness in a family is a misfortune. It is usually nobody's fault; no one is responsible for it. But we face choices about how we will respond to this misfortune. That's where the responsibility comes in and fault can arise. Those of us with families and loved ones always have a duty not to make selfish or self-centered decisions about our lives. We have a responsibility to try to protect the lives of loved ones from serious threats or greatly impoverished quality, certainly an obligation not to make choices that will jeopardize or seriously compromise their futures. Often, it would be wrong to do just what we want or just what is best for ourselves; we should choose in light of what is best for all concerned. That is our duty in sickness as well as in health. It is out of these responsibilities that a duty to die can develop.

I am not advocating a crass, quasi-economic conception of burdens and benefits, nor a shallow, hedonistic view of life. Given a suitably rich understanding of benefits, family members sometimes do benefit from suffering through the long illness of a loved one. Caring for the sick or aged can foster growth, even as it makes daily life immeasurably harder and the prospects for the future much bleaker. Chronic illness or a drawn-out death can also pull a family together, making the care for each other stronger and more evident. If my loved ones are truly benefiting from coping with my illness or debility, I have no duty to die based on burdens to them.

But it would be irresponsible to blithely assume that this always happens, that it will happen in my family, or that it will be the fault of my family if they cannot manage to turn my illness into a positive experience. Perhaps the opposite is more common: A hospital chaplain once told me that he could not think of a single case in which a family was strengthened or brought together by what happened at the hospital.

Our families and loved ones also have obligations, of course—they have the responsibility to stand by us and to support us through debilitating illness and death. They must be prepared to make significant sacrifices to respond to an illness in the family. I am far from denying that. Most of us are aware of this responsibility and most families meet it rather well. In fact, families deliver more than 80 percent of the long-term care in this country, almost always at great personal cost. Most of us who are a part of a family can expect to be sustained in our time of need by family members and those who love us.

But most discussions of an illness in the family sound as if responsibility were a one-way street. It is not, of course. When we become seriously ill or debilitated, we too may have to make sacrifices. To think that my loved ones must bear whatever burdens my illness, debility, or dying process might impose upon them is to reduce them to means to my well-being. And that would be immoral. Family solidarity, altruism, bearing the burden of a loved one's misfortune, and loyalty are all important virtues of families, as well. But they are all also two-way streets.

OBJECTIONS TO A DUTY TO DIE

To my mind, the most serious objections to the idea of a duty to die lie in the effects on my loved ones of ending my life. But to most others, the important objections have little or nothing to do with family and loved ones. Perhaps the most common objections are: (1) There is a higher duty that always takes precedence over a duty to die; (2) a duty to end one's own life would be incompatible with a recognition of human dignity or the intrinsic value of a person; and (3) seriously ill, debilitated, or dying people are already bearing the harshest burdens and so it would be wrong to ask them to bear the additional burden of ending their own lives.

These are all important objections; all deserve a thorough discussion. Here I will only be able to suggest some moral counterweights—ideas that might provide the basis for an argument that these objections do not always preclude a duty to die.

An example of the first line of argument would be the claim that a duty to God, the giver of life, forbids that anyone take her own life. It could be argued that this duty always supersedes whatever obligations we might have to our families. But what convinces us that we always have such a religious duty in the first place? And what guarantees that it always supersedes our obligations to try to protect our loved ones?

Certainly, the view that death is the ultimate evil cannot be squared with Christian theology. It does not reflect the actions of Jesus or those of his early followers. Nor is it clear that the belief that life is sacred requires that we never take it. There are other theological possibilities.[6] In any case, most of us—bioethicists, physicians, and patients alike—do not subscribe to the view that we have an obligation to preserve human life as long as possible. But if not, surely we ought to agree that I may legitimately end my life for other-regarding reasons, not just for self-regarding reasons.

Secondly, religious considerations aside, the claim could be made that an obligation to end one's own life would be incompatible with human dignity or would embody a failure to recognize the intrinsic value of a person. But I do not see that in thinking I had a duty to die I would necessarily be failing to respect myself or to appreciate my dignity or worth. Nor would I necessarily be failing to respect you in thinking that you had a similar duty. There is surely also a sense in which we fail to respect ourselves if in the face of illness or death, we stoop to choosing just what is best for ourselves. Indeed, Kant held that the very core of human dignity is the ability to act on a self-imposed moral law, regardless of whether it is in our interest to do so.[7] We shall return to the notion of human dignity.

A third objection appeals to the relative weight of burdens and thus, ultimately, to considerations of fairness or justice. The burdens that an illness creates for the family could not possibly be great enough to justify an obligation to end one's life—the sacrifice of life itself would be a far greater burden than any involved in caring for a chronically ill family member.

But is this true? Consider the following case:

> An 87-year-old woman was dying of congestive heart failure. Her APACHE score predicted that she had less than a 50 percent chance to live for another six months. She was lucid, assertive, and terrified of death. She very much wanted to live and kept opting for rehospitalization and the most aggressive lifeprolonging treatment possible. That treatment successfully prolonged her life (though with increasing debility) for nearly 2 years. Her 55-year-old daughter was her only remaining family, her caregiver, and the main source of her financial support. The daughter duly cared for her mother. But before her mother died, her illness had cost the daughter all of her savings, her home, her job, and her career.

This is by no means an uncommon sort of case. Thousands of similar cases occur each year. Now, ask yourself which is the greater burden:

> a. To lose a 50 percent chance of six more months of life at age 87?
> b. To lose all your savings, your home, and your career at age 55?

Which burden would you prefer to bear? Do we really believe the former is the greater burden? Would even the dying mother say that (a) is the greater burden? Or has she been encouraged to believe that the burdens of (b) are somehow morally irrelevant to her choices?

I think most of us would quickly agree that (b) is a greater burden. That is the evil we would more hope to avoid in our lives. If we are tempted to say that the mother's disease and impending death are the greater evil, I believe it is because we are taking a "slice of time" perspective rather than a "lifetime perspective."[8] But surely the lifetime perspective is the appropriate perspective when weighing burdens. If (b) is the greater burden, then we must admit that we have been promulgating an ethics that advocates imposing greater burdens on some people in order to provide smaller benefits for others just because they are ill and thus gain our professional attention and advocacy.

A whole range of cases like this one could easily be generated. In some, the answer about which burden is greater will not be clear. But in many it is. Death—or ending your own life—is simply not the greatest evil or the greatest burden.

This point does not depend on a utilitarian calculus. Even if death were the greatest burden (thus disposing of any simple utilitarian argument), serious questions would remain about the moral justifiability of choosing to impose crushing burdens on loved ones in order to avoid having to bear this burden oneself. The fact that I suffer greater burdens than others in my family does not license me simply to choose what I want for myself, nor does it necessarily release me from a responsibility to try to protect the quality of their lives.

I can readily imagine that, through cowardice, rationalization, or failure of resolve, I will fail in this obligation to protect my loved ones. If so, I think I would need to be excused or forgiven for what I did. But I cannot imagine it would be morally permissible for me to ruin the rest of my partner's life to sustain mine or to cut off my sons' careers, impoverish them, or compromise the quality of their children's lives simply because I wish to live a little longer. This is what leads me to believe in a duty to die.

Who Has a Duty to Die?

Suppose, then, that there can be a duty to die. Who has a duty to die? And when? To my mind, these are the right questions, the questions we should be asking. Many of us may one day badly need answers to just these questions.

But I cannot supply answers here, for two reasons. In the first place, answers will have to be very particular and contextual. Our concrete duties are often situated, defined in part by the myriad details of our circumstances, histories, and relationships. Though there may be principles that apply to a wide range of cases and some cases that yield pretty straightforward answers, there will also be many situations in which it is very difficult to discern whether one has a duty to die. If nothing else, it will often be very difficult to predict how one's family will bear up under the weight of the burdens that a protracted illness would impose on them. Momentous decisions will often have to be made under conditions of great uncertainty.

Second and perhaps even more importantly, I believe that those of us with family and loved ones should not define our duties unilat-

erally, especially not a decision about a duty to die. It would be isolating and distancing for me to decide without consulting them what
is too much of a burden for my loved ones to bear. That way of deciding about my moral duties is not only atomistic, it also treats my family and loved ones paternalistically. They must be allowed to speak for
themselves about the burdens my life imposes on them and how they
feel about bearing those burdens.

Some may object that it would be wrong to put a loved one in a
position of having to say, in effect, "You should end your life because
caring for you is too hard on me and the rest of the family." Not only
will it be almost impossible to say something like that to someone
you love, it will carry with it a heavy load of guilt. On this view, you
should decide by yourself whether you have a duty to die and
approach your loved ones only after you have made up your mind to
say good-bye to them. Your family could then try to change your
mind, but the tremendous weight of moral decision would be lifted
from their shoulders.

Perhaps so. But I believe in family decisions. Important decisions
for those whose lives are interwoven should be made together, in a
family discussion. Granted, a conversation about whether I have a
duty to die would be a tremendously difficult conversation. The
temptations to be dishonest could be enormous. Nevertheless, if I am
contemplating a duty to die, my family and I should, if possible, have
just such an agonizing discussion. It will act as a check on the information, perceptions, and reasoning of all of us. But even more importantly, it affirms our connectedness at a critical juncture in our lives
and our life together. Honest talk about difficult matters almost
always strengthens relationships.

However, many families seem unable to talk about death at all,
much less a duty to die. Certainly most families could not have this
discussion all at once, in one sitting. It might well take a number of
discussions to be able to approach this topic. But even if talking about
death is impossible, there are always behavioral clues—about your
caregiver's tiredness, physical condition, health, prevailing mood,
anxiety, financial concerns, outlook, overall well-being, and so on.
And families unable to talk about death can often talk about how the
caregiver is feeling, about finances, about tensions within the family
resulting from the illness, about concerns for the future. Deciding
whether you have a duty to die based on these behavioral clues and
conversation about them honors your relationships better than

deciding on your own about how burdensome you and your care must be.

I cannot say when someone has a duty to die. Still, I can suggest a few features of one's illness, history, and circumstances that make it more likely that one has a duty to die. I present them here without much elaboration or explanation.

1. A duty to die is more likely when continuing to live will impose significant burden—emotional burdens, extensive caregiving, destruction of life plans, and, yes, financial hardship—on your family and loved ones. This is the fundamental insight underlying a duty to die.

2. A duty to die becomes greater as you grow older. As we age, we will be giving up less by giving up our lives, if only because we will sacrifice fewer remaining years of life and a smaller portion of our life plans. After all, it's not as if we would be immortal and live forever if we could just manage to avoid a duty to die. To have reached the age of, say, 75 or 80 years without being ready to die is itself a moral failing, the sign of a life out of touch with life's basic realities.[9]

3. A duty to die is more likely when you have already lived a full and rich life. You have already had a full share of the good things life offers.

4. There is greater duty to die if your loved ones' lives have already been difficult or impoverished, if they have had only a small share of the good things that life has to offer (especially if through no fault of their own).

5. A duty to die is more likely when your loved ones have already made great contributions—perhaps even sacrifices—to make your life a good one. Especially if you have not made similar sacrifices for their well-being or for the well-being of other members of your family.

6. To the extent that you can make a good adjustment to your illness or handicapping condition, there is less likely to be a duty to die. A good adjustment means that smaller sacrifices will be required of loved ones and there is more compensating interaction for them. Still, we must also recognize that some diseases—Alzheimer or Huntington chorea—will eventually take their toll on your loved ones no matter how courageously, resolutely, even cheerfully you manage to face that illness.

7. There is less likely to be a duty to die if you can still make significant

contributions to the lives of others, especially your family. The burdens to family members are not only or even primarily financial, neither are the contributions to them. However, the old and those who have terminal illnesses must also bear in mind that the loss their family members will feel when they die cannot be avoided, only postponed.

8. A duty to die is more likely when the part of you that is loved will soon be gone or seriously compromised. Or when you soon will no longer be capable of giving love. Part of the horror of dementing disease is that it destroys the capacity to nurture and sustain relationships, taking away a person's agency and the emotions that bind her to others.

9. There is a greater duty to die to the extent that you have lived a relatively lavish lifestyle instead of saving for illness or old age. Like most upper middle-class Americans, I could easily have saved more. It is a greater wrong to come to your family for assistance if your need is the result of having chosen leisure or a spendthrift lifestyle. I may eventually have to face the moral consequences of decisions I am now making.

These, then, are some of the considerations that give shape and definition to the duty to die. If we can agree that these considerations are all relevant, we can see that the correct course of action will often be difficult to discern. A decision about when I should end my life will sometimes prove to be every bit as difficult as the decision about whether I want treatment for myself.

Can the Incompetent Have a Duty to Die?

Severe mental deterioration springs readily to mind as one of the situations in which I believe I could have a duty to die. But can incompetent people have duties at all? We can have moral duties we do not recognize or acknowledge, including duties that we never recognized. But can we have duties we are unable to recognize? Duties when we are unable to understand the concept of morality at all? If so, do others have a moral obligation to help us carry out this duty? These are extremely difficult theoretical questions. The reach of moral agency is severely strained by mental incompetence.

I am tempted to simply bypass the entire question by saying that I am talking only about competent persons. But the idea of a duty to die clearly raises the specter of one person claiming that another—

who cannot speak for herself—has such a duty. So I need to say that I can make no sense of the claim that someone has a duty to die if the person has never been able to understand moral obligation at all. To my mind, only those who were formerly capable of making moral decisions could have such a duty.

But the case of formerly competent persons is almost as troubling. Perhaps we should simply stipulate that no incompetent person can have a duty to die, not even if she affirmed belief in such a duty in an advance directive. If we take the view that formerly competent people may have such a duty, we should surely exercise extreme caution when claiming a formerly competent person would have acknowledged a duty to die or that any formerly competent person has an unacknowledged duty to die. Moral dangers loom regardless of which way we decide to resolve such issues.

But for me personally, very urgent practical matters turn on their resolution. If a formerly competent person can no longer have a duty to die (or if other people are not likely to help her carry out this duty), I believe that my obligation may be to die while I am still competent, before I become unable to make and carry out that decision for myself. Surely it would be irresponsible to evade my moral duties by temporizing until I escape into incompetence. And so I must die sooner than I otherwise would have to. On the other hand, if I could count on others to end my life after I become incompetent, I might be able to fulfill my responsibilities while also living out all my competent or semicompetent days. Given our society's reluctance to permit physicians, let alone family members, to perform aid-in-dying, I believe I may well have a duty to end my life when I can see mental incapacity on the horizon.

There is also the very real problem of sudden incompetence—due to a serious stroke or automobile accident, for example. For me, that is the real nightmare. If I suddenly become incompetent, I will fall into the hands of a medical-legal system that will conscientiously disregard my moral beliefs and do what is best for me, regardless of the consequences for my loved ones. And that is not at all what I would have wanted!

Social Policies and a Duty to Die

The claim that there is a duty to die will seem to some a misplaced response to social negligence. If our society were providing for the debilitated, the chronically ill, and the elderly as it should be, there would be only very rare cases of a duty to die. On this view, I am asking the sick and debilitated to step in and accept responsibility because society is derelict in its responsibility to provide for the incapacitated.

This much is surely true: There are a number of social policies we could pursue that would dramatically reduce the incidence of such a duty. Most obviously, we could decide to pay for facilities that provided excellent longterm care (not just health care!) for all chronically ill, debilitated, mentally ill, or demented people in this country. We probably could still afford to do this. If we did, sick, debilitated, and dying people might still be morally required to make sacrifices for their families. I might, for example, have a duty to forgo personal care by a family member who knows me and really does care for me. But these sacrifices would only rarely include the sacrifice of life itself. The duty to die would then be virtually eliminated.

I cannot claim to know whether in some abstract sense a society like ours should provide care for all who are chronically ill or debilitated. But the fact is that we Americans seem to be unwilling to pay for this kind of long-term care, except for ourselves and our own. In fact, we are moving in precisely the opposite direction—we are trying to shift the burdens of caring for the seriously and chronically ill onto families in order to save costs for our health care system. As we shift the burdens of care onto families, we also dramatically increase the number of Americans who will have a duty to die. I must not, then, live my life and make my plans on the assumption that social institutions will protect my family from my infirmity and debility. To do so would be irresponsible. More likely, it will be up to me to protect my loved ones.

A Duty to Die and the Meaning of Life

A duty to die seems very harsh, and often it would be. It is one of the tragedies of our lives that someone who wants very much to live can nevertheless have a duty to die. It is both tragic and ironic that it is precisely the very real good of family and loved ones that gives rise to this duty. Indeed, the genuine love, closeness, and supportiveness of family members is a major source of this duty: we could not be such a burden if they did not care for us. Finally, there is deep irony in the fact that the very successes of our life-prolonging medicine help to create a widespread duty to die. We do not live in such a happy world that we can avoid such tragedies and ironies. We ought not to close our eyes to this reality or pretend that it just doesn't exist. We ought not to minimize the tragedy in any way.

And yet, a duty to die will not always be as harsh as we might assume. If I love my family, I will want to protect them and their lives. I will want not to make choices that compromise their futures. Indeed, I can easily imagine that I might want to avoid compromising their lives more than I would want anything else. I must also admit that I am not necessarily giving up so much in giving up my life: the conditions that give rise to a duty to die would usually already have compromised the quality of the life I am required to end. In any case, I personally must confess that at age 56, I have already lived a very good life, albeit not yet nearly as long a life as I would like to have.

We fear death too much. Our fear of death has lead to a massive assault on it. We still crave virtually any life-prolonging technology that we might conceivably be able to produce. We still too often feel morally impelled to prolong life—virtually any form of life—as long as possible. As if the best death is the one that can be put off longest.

We do not even ask about meaning in death, so busy are we with trying to postpone it. But we will not conquer death by one day developing a technology so magnificent that no one will have to die. Nor can we conquer death by postponing it ever longer. We can conquer death only by finding meaning in it.

Although the existence of a duty to die does not hinge on this, recognizing such a duty would go some way toward recovering meaning in death. Paradoxically, it would restore dignity to those who are seriously ill or dying. It would also reaffirm the connections required to give life (and death) meaning. I close now with a few words about both of these points.

First, recognizing a duty to die affirms my agency and also my moral agency. I can still do things that make an important difference in the lives of my loved ones. Moreover, the fact that I still have responsibilities keeps me within the community of moral agents. My illness or debility has not reduced me to a mere moral patient (to use the language of the philosophers). Though it may not be the whole story, surely Kant was onto something important when he claimed that human dignity rests on the capacity for moral agency within a community of those who respect the demands of morality.

By contrast, surely there is something deeply insulting in a medicine and an ethic that would ask only what I want (or would have wanted) when I become ill. To treat me as if I had no moral responsibilities when I am ill or debilitated implies that my condition has rendered me morally incompetent. Only small children, the demented or insane, and those totally lacking in the capacity to act are free from moral duties. There is dignity, then, and a kind of meaning in moral agency, even as it forces extremely difficult decisions upon us.

Second, recovering meaning in death requires an affirmation of connections. If I end my life to spare the futures of my loved ones, I testify in my death that I am connected to them. It is because I love and care for precisely these people (and I know they care for me) that I wish not to be such a burden to them. By contrast, a life in which I am free to choose whatever I want for myself is a life unconnected to others. A bioethics that would treat me as if I had no serious moral responsibilities does what it can to marginalize, weaken, or even destroy my connections with others.

But life without connection is meaningless. The individualistic fantasy, though occasionally liberating, is deeply destructive. When life is good and vitality seems unending, life itself and life lived for yourself may seem quite sufficient. But if not life, certainly death without connection is meaningless. If you are only for yourself, all you have to care about as your life draws to a close is yourself and your life. Everything you care about will then perish in your death. And that—the end of everything you care about—is precisely the total collapse of meaning. We can, then, find meaning in death only through a sense of connection with something that will survive our death.

This need not be connections with other people. Some people are deeply tied to land (for example, the family farm), to nature, or to a transcendent reality. But for most of us, the connections that sustain us are to other people. In the full bloom of life, we are connected to others in many ways—through work, profession, neighborhood, country, shared faith and worship, common leisure pursuits, friendship. Even the guru meditating in isolation on his mountain top is connected to a long tradition of people united by the same religious quest.

But as we age or when we become chronically ill, connections with other people usually become much more restricted. Often, only ties with family and close friends remain and remain important to us. Moreover, for many of us, other connections just don't go deep enough. As Paul Tsongas has reminded us, "When it comes time to

134

die, no one says, 'I wish I had spent more time at the office.'"

If I am correct, death is so difficult for us partly because our sense of community is so weak. Death seems to wipe out everything when we can't fit it into the lives of those who live on. A death motivated by the desire to spare the futures of my loved ones might well be a better death for me than the one I would get as a result of opting to continue my life as long as there is any pleasure in it for me. Pleasure is nice, but it is meaning that matters.

I don't know about others, but these reflections have helped me. I am now more at peace about facing a duty to die. Ending my own life if duty required might still be difficult. But for me, a far greater horror would be dying all alone or stealing the futures of my loved ones in order to buy a little more time for myself. I hope that if the time comes when I have a duty to die, I will recognize it, encourage my loved ones to recognize it too, and carry it out bravely.

ACKNOWLEDGMENTS

I wish to thank Mary English, Hilde Nelson, Jim Bennett, Tom Townsend, the members of the Philosophy Department at East Tennessee State University, and anonymous reviewers of the Report for many helpful comments on earlier versions of this paper. In this paper, I draw on material in John Hardwig, "Dying at the Right Time; Reflections on (Un)Assisted Suicide." *Practical Ethics*. Ed. H. LaFollette. London: Blackwell, 1996, with permission.

NOTES

1. Given the importance of relationships in my thinking, "responsibility"—rooted as it is in "respond"—would perhaps be the most appropriate word. Nevertheless, I often use "duty" despite its legalistic overtones, because Lamm's famous statement has given the expression "duty to die" a certain familiarity. But I intend no implication that there is a law that grounds this duty, nor that someone has a right corresponding to it.

2. For a discussion of the Oates case, see Tom L. Beauchamp, "What Is Suicide?" *Ethical Issues in Death and Dying*. Eds. Tom L. Beauchamp and Seymour Perlin. Englewood Cliffs, NJ: Prentice-Hall, 1978.

3. Most bioethicists advocate a "patient-centered ethics"—an ethics which claims only the patient's interests should be considered in making medical treatment decisions. Most health care professionals have been trained to accept this ethic and to see themselves as patient advocates. For arguments that a patient-centered ethics should be replaced by a family-centered ethics, see John Hardwig, "What About the Family?" *Hastings Center Report* 20.2 (1990): 5–10; Hilde L. Nelson, and James L. Nelson. *The Patient in the Family*. New York: Routledge, 1995.

4. A good account of the burdens of caregiving can be found in Elaine Brody, *Women in the Middle: Their Parent-Care Years.* New York: Springer, 1990. Perhaps the best article-length account of these burdens is Daniel Callahan, "Families as Caregivers; the Limits of Morality." *Aging and Ethics: Philosophical Problems in Gerontology.* Ed. Nancy Jecker. Totowa, NJ: Humana Press, 1991.

5. Kenneth E. Covinsky, et al. "The Impact of Serious Illness on Patients' Families," *Journal of the American Medical Association* 272 (1994): 1839–44.

6. Larry Churchill, for example, believes that Christian ethics takes us far beyond my present position: "Christian doctrines of stewardship prohibit the extension of one's own life at a great cost to the neighbor . . . and such a gesture should not appear to us a sacrifice, but as the ordinary virtue entailed by a just, social conscience." Larry Churchill, *Rationing Health Care in America.* South Bend, IN:/ Notre Dame UP, 1988), 112.

7. Kant, as is well known, was opposed to suicide. But he was arguing against taking your life out of self-interested motives. It is not clear that Kant would or we should consider taking your life out of a sense of duty to be wrong. See Hilde L. Nelson, "Death with Kantian Dignity:/," *Journal of Clinical Ethics* 7 (1996): 215–21.

8. Obviously, I owe this distinction to Norman Daniels. Norman Daniels, *Am I My Parents' Keeper? An Essay on Justice Between the Young and the Old.* New York: Oxford UP, 1988. Just as obviously, Daniels is not committed to my use of it here.

9. Daniel Callahan, *The Troubled Dream of Life.* New York: Simon & Schuster, 1993.

Commentaries on "Is There a Duty to Die?"

Duty to Die?
Nat Hentoff

While he was governor of Colorado, Richard Lamm became, for a time, a troubling national presence, not as a result of his politics but because of the challenge he issued to the citizenry in every state. At an autumnal age, he said, it is a moral responsibility to make room for the young. As leaves fall from the trees in the fall, so old people have a duty to die.

The governor and I were asked to debate this proposition at Pennsylvania State University. When we arrived at the hotel in the afternoon, he urgently asked the desk clerk if there was a gym nearby where he could have his customary workout. It occurred to me that he wanted to delay the day, as best he could, when his own leaves would fall.

As a consequence of the current national debate on physician-assisted suicide, its opponents have predicted that if assisted suicide is legalized, people whose illnesses are costly and long-term may be convinced they have a duty to die. Feeling guilty because of the burden they have become to their families, they—with suicide now approved by society—may ask their doctors to help them die.

Now, in certain bioethical circles, the morality of dying as a utilitarian imperative is being advanced. Those who mocked Gov. Lamm's advice to go responsibly into the good night may have been premature.

The *Hastings Center Report* is one of the more respected journals dealing with the nature of human nature and medical ethics. The leading article on the cover of its March/April issue is John Hardwig's

"Is There a Duty to Die?" The author teaches medical ethics and social political philosophy at East Tennessee State University.

At the start, Hardwig declares that, "modern medicine and an individualistic culture have seduced many [into believing] that they have a right to health care and a right to live, despite the burdens and costs to our families and society."

Hardwig recognizes that there already is a legal right to refuse life-prolonging medical treatment. But, he claims, "a duty to die can go well beyond that. . . . There may be a fairly common responsibility to end one's life in the absence of any terminal illness." Indeed, "there can be a duty to die even when one would prefer to live."

After all, "the lives of our loved ones can be seriously compromised by caring for us. . . . There is a sense in which we fail to respect ourselves if in the face of illness or death, we stoop to choosing just what is best for ourselves."

Years ago, Michigan University law professor Yale Kamisar predicted that with the coming of assisted suicide, precisely this kind of argument could well persuade vulnerable patients to let themselves slip into eternity—rather than remain a burden.

Hardwig also makes the stern point that as we grow older, the duty to die becomes more compelling because "we will be giving up less . . . we will sacrifice fewer remaining years of life." (Perhaps copies of Walter Huston singing "September Song" may ease the way.)

Hardwig presses on: "To have reached the age of, say, 75 or 80 years without being ready to die is itself a moral failing, the sign of a life out of touch with life's basic realities."

Will octogenarians who are not ready to die be publicly shamed as the moral community shuns them?

There is another criterion for being ready to join the falling leaves in autumn. "A duty to die," says Hardwig, "is more likely when you have already lived a rich and full life. You have already had a full share of the good things life offers." I assume that the chronically poor as well as long-term prisoners are given compensatory time to stay alive.

But there is a way out for most of the rest of us. If, Hardwig says, the society is willing to "pay for facilities that provide excellent long-term care (not just health care) for all chronically ill, debilitated, mentally ill or demented people in this country . . . the duty to die would then be virtually eliminated."

Hardwig, however, is a realist: "We Americans seem to be unwilling to pay for this kind of long-term care, except for ourselves and our own." There will be no escaping, then, a duty to die, provided, says Hardwig, we have the courage to die in order to protect our loved ones from the costs, financially and emotionally, of our staying on.

John Hardwig is not alone. I have heard doctors say that certain patients, taking up expensive space in a hospital, have a duty to die because they will never be able to walk out of the hospital. Dr. Jack Kevorkian is his own kind of ethicist, but if his bedside manner were not so startling, he would be seen as not far from the current ready-to-die mainstream.

John Hardwig says, "We fear death too much." My sense is we do not fear bioethicists enough.

OUR BURDEN UPON OTHERS: A RESPONSE TO JOHN HARDWIG
Daniel Callahan

Ever since I first read John Hardwig's article on a duty to die, I have tried to find a way to take seriously his argument. I have profited from other articles he has written, typically marked by insight and good sense. His sustained effort to find a richer ethic than the reigning narcissistic individualism is an important contribution to our common life. His moral struggle with the issue he raises in this article strikes me as clearly worthy of our respect and attention. And since I have, in some of my own writings relevant to his topic, been subject to considerable opprobrium, I can empathize with someone trying to make a case that goes against the cultural grain.

Even so, I think he is fundamentally wrong in this instance. His "duty to die" seems to me a threat to families and the community, not a benefit, and his ideas about moral obligation, human dignity, and death are likely to do far more harm than good. I wish I could find something nice to say for his argument. I can't.

This might seem surprising since I have advanced an argument in some of my own writing that might seem relevant to, and supportive of, his claim. In *Setting Limits: Medical Goals in an Aging Society*, I tried to make the case that, while we have a strong societal obligation to provide health care for the old, it is not an unlimited obligation. At some point in the future, when the baby-boom generation retires, it may be necessary to limit expensive life-extending treatment of the elderly using age itself as the criterion for limitation. The justification for doing so is the unfair burden that unlimited care for the elderly would place upon a younger generation. An age-based rationing, I contended, could be both fair and respectful of the dignity of the old (provided that they had been part of a democratic process approving such rationing—it would have to be adopted only with their consent). That was not a popular proposal. "Social euthanasia" was the way one critic characterized it.

In making that argument, I explicitly rejected a "duty to die." There is a difference of great importance between a duty to die and a duty to accept a limitation of resources which will increase the risk of death, even significantly. In the former case, the aim is to be dead by (presumably) suicide if that is what it takes. In the latter case, by contrast, we are being asked to run a risk of death, but death by disease rather than by our own hand.

The ethics of just warfare offers a pertinent analogy here. Young people can be drafted to come to the defense of their society (assuming it *is* a just war) and society can demand that they put themselves at risk of death. But no theory of just war holds that there is a duty to die or to be killed for the sake of others. Soldiers who throw themselves upon grenades to save the lives of their comrades are given medals for conduct "above and beyond the call of duty." We ought to be willing to risk an earlier death in old age for the sake of others, but we have no duty to kill ourselves for others.

Why is there no such duty? I move now to Hardwig's contention. I will offer four considerations that I believe together show that there can be no duty to die and the harmful consequences that would result should we invent such a duty. I will try to show (1) that the logic of a duty claim carries with it untoward entailments, none of which are acceptable; (2) that it would be nightmarish in practice for families and individuals to try to live out (so to speak) such a duty; (3) that a duty to die for the sake of others would be destructive of families; and (4) that Hardwig's notion of human dignity bleaches that concept of serious weight.

1. *The logic of a duty to die.* In ordinary usage, a "duty" of one person to do something with respect to another person (or group) entails a right on the part of that other person to demand that the duty be carried out. One person's duty to relieve a burden upon another is that other person's right to have that burden lifted. But if that is so, there is a problem: who decides if the burden is insupportable, the person supposedly burdened or the person who believes he is being a burden? The former would seem to be in a far better position to make

that judgment than the latter, in which case he can demand that the other commit suicide, whether that person wants to or not—for it is his duty not to be a burden and the right of the other person to demand that of him. The logic of that relationship between duty and rights opens the door to family tyranny.

It would also seem true that a duty to die entails someone else's right to kill us. For if in fact we are a burden, and have no right to be that, then the person whom we are burdening should be free to kill us. Our duty to die seems to require someone else's right to kill us if we fail to recognize or accept our duty. Closely related to that logic is the entailment that we owe our death to our family if we are a burden upon them; it becomes their right to demand that of us. Hardwig has, moreover, said that there can be a "fairly common responsibility to end one's life in the absence of any terminal illness at all" if that life is a family burden. That of course will nicely allow a claim upon the disabled and dependent to relieve us of any false feelings that we have a duty to care for them; and also, should they not see the light about *their* duty, the right to kill them if they refuse to respect our right to demand they do their duty.

In none of these cases will it do to say that there must always be competence and consent on the part of the person who has a duty to die. For if there is a serious "duty," then we have a right to insist that it be acted upon. It makes no sense to talk of a voluntary duty, since duties have strong moral standings, much more than just *feeling* one has a duty. Parents have a duty to raise their children well and safely, and we legally and morally hold them to that duty whether they accept it or not. A serious notion of a "duty to die" would seem, as Hardwig develops it, no less stringent or impersonal in its moral requirements.

Consent to duty here is beside the point. This principle, by the way, would also seem to obviate Hardwig's desire to exempt the incompetent from the duty. If an incompetent person is a burden, he is a burden. If the aim is to assist a family, then it is hard to see why the incompetence of a family member destroys that family's right to be relieved of the burden. Should wealthy, but incompetent, fathers be relieved of their duty to support their children on the grounds of their incompetence? The fact that such a person "could not understand moral obligation at all" (to use Hardwig's expression) would hardly deprive a court of the right to garnish money from his bank account to satisfy the rights (and needs) of his children.

2. *Family circle.* Hardwig does not use his imagination as much as he might in trying to envision what it would be like for families to negotiate a duty to die. Much suffering is subjective, a function of personal values and particular circumstances. A dying or otherwise burdensome person cared for by a career-minded person will probably be more of a burden than someone happier to be a caregiver. Some people seem more naturally giving and self-sacrificial than others; some people can't stand helping others. But is a duty to die to depend upon the emotional vagaries and differential values of caregivers? What happens if a family is divided, some feeling unburdened and others feeling much put upon? Whose judgment will count?

The same subjectivity will come into play with the sick person. Here again people range along a continuum, some quite willing to burden others, some utterly unwilling. The values and life experience of the sick person will and must come into play. But can a "duty to die" be based upon that kind of continuum? Those happy to burden others will feel no duty to die to relieve those they burden, and they are hardly like to give their consent to die. Are they thereby exempt from the duty, while those who can't stand the thought of burdening others are bound by it?

I am simply of course raising problems here, but they are impossible to overlook. At the least, families will be open to highly unpleasant second-guessing, guilt, uncertainty, and confusion. Their trust of each other will be put to a supreme test, and it is hard to see how that trust could endure in many imaginable cases. Think only about a situation where a family member believed and said that the sick person had a duty to die, that is, to kill herself. If the sick person did not believe that, how could she ever trust the motives of those who had informed her of her duty to get out of their lives? Hardwig seems to want a kind of tough love about such problems, as if they must be faced up to regardless of the unhappiness raising them might create. That seems to me potentially cruel.

3. *Sustaining families.* I have already tried to show that the practical problems and puzzles that a duty-to-die morality would pose for families would themselves be destructive. Now I want to make a still stronger case: a family that would let one of their members kill himself for their benefit would wreak havoc with the very meaning of "family." If not in its literal denotative sense, "family" has come to mean connotatively a "haven in a heartless world," to use the title of a book by Christopher Lasch. Robert Frost caught the same flavor

when he wrote in his poem "The Death of the Hired Man" that "home is the place where, when you have to go there/They have to take you in." I would put it this way: the family should be that place where a cost-benefit calculus must be left outside the door, where we bear each other's burdens come what may. Where Frost says of the "home" (which I take to be the family) that "They have to take you in," I would want to add "and they won't throw you out" as long as it is not your fault that you have imposed yourself upon their love and devotion.

Hardwig talks about all this in a strange way: "To think that my loved one must bear whatever burdens my illness, debility, or dying process might impose upon them is to reduce them to means to my well-being." This is a distortion of the Kantian principle that people should be treated as ends only, never as means. The sick or dying person has not in any way deliberately "imposed" himself on anyone. He did not choose his illness or (usually) the social circumstance of his illness that has imposed itself upon his family. He did not, in short, choose them to be means to his end. He had no choice about the matter, and it would seem gratuitous in the extreme to accuse him of a sin of omission for refusing to try, by way of death, to change that situation.

It would in fact be a family that responded to some supposed duty of a dependent, burdensome sick person to die that would be violating the Kantian maxim. For they would, with his collusion, choose his death as a means to *their* ends, that of being free of the trouble of caring for him. But where he had no choice about the medical condition that brought him to depend upon his family, they will have knowingly and deliberately allowed him to sacrifice himself for their ends if they approve of, and abet, his death.

If even societies in the throes of war and imminent destruction cannot invoke a duty to die among its defenders, it is hard to see how the good of the family can lead to that conclusion. Families in which their members were ready to kill themselves for some greater familial good, and to allow each other to acquiesce in death for that reason, would in principle be treating each other as dispensable and disposable once they got too much in the way.

I would suggest that the very meaning of family in the wider sense I invoked above makes such a calculation not only improper but also morally unthinkable. Instead of the family being a "haven in a heartless world" it would *become* that heartless world in microcosm, counting utiles of burden and trouble—and all the worse for being dressed up in the sentimental language of decency and self-sacrifice. Family life is a "two-way" street, but for me this means that I should be willing both to take up the burden of caring for another come what may and be no less willing to be a burden to another. It is indeed, as Hardwig writes, tragic "that my loved ones would be much better off . . . if I were dead." But it would escalate a tragedy to an evil to praise a situation where their death in such circumstances was countenanced (by agreeing to their chosen death) and they themselves praised for thinking they had a duty to die.

4. *Human dignity.* Hardwig tells us at the end of his article that he is now "more at peace about facing a duty to die." But if so, it strikes me as a false peace, the kind that makes us feel good but does not do good. For all the reasons noted above, it will introduce a latent and deadly virus into his future family life. It will also serve to perpetuate one of the great moral errors of the late 20th century: that moral agency confers human dignity.

One passage nicely catches that whole sad story. "Recognizing a duty to die," Hardwig writes, "affirms my agency and also my moral agency. I can still do things that make an important difference in the lives of my loved ones. Moreover, the fact that I can still have responsibilities keeps me within the community of moral agents. . . . There is dignity, then, and a kind of meaning in moral agency, even as it forces extremely difficult decisions upon us." The trouble with all this is twofold. First, it implies that only a decision to die would count as moral agency, not a decision to bear the illness and to allow oneself to be dependent upon one's family. But if Hardwig believes we have a choice here, either choice can express moral agency. Second, he implies that there is something selfish about those who choose to endure their illness and also endure, with it, the difficulties they bring upon their families. Dignity, he says, resides only in a choice to relieve a family of those difficulties. Is he then saying that the helpless, the demented, children, and others who cannot act, who lack the ability to make moral choices have forfeited an honorable, dignified place in the community or the family? Or that those who fail to perceive their duty to die, and thus to act properly, have betrayed the moral community and forfeited their own dignity?

I doubt that Hardwig would want to say this, but by tying moral agency in so closely with human dignity, and then further stipulating a choice to die as an exalted expression of agency, he opens himself up to just that criticism. He also ignores the possibility that there can be dignity in the choice of families that bear their misfortune, even when it is destructive of their lives. Does not their moral agency count? Is it not also the case that living a moral life can at times be destructive of our worldly aims? If it can be a legitimate expression of moral agency to care for a sick person at high personal cost, something good to do, then it is hard to see why it would be wrong for the sick person to accept that care; and it is imaginable that, in some cases, it would be wrong to deprive a family of that moral possibility if they chose to accept it.

I simply lay out moral possibilities here, if only to show that the moral universe offers far more dignity-affirming choices and circumstances than Hardwig imagines. There can, in the end, be no morally sensible "duty to die." It would almost certainly be destructive of family bonds and trust and legitimate even more deeply a thin, almost trivialized meaning of human dignity. A duty to die becomes someone else's claim of their right that I die. My willingness to make a noble sacrifice will all too easily tempt some, for their ends, to encourage me on to death. Giving them the language of duty to work with—my duty, not theirs—will make them feel all the better for trying. After all, they will only be asking me to give them that which I owe them anyway, for what else is duty all about than giving others what is their due?

I hope Hardwig will spare his family that temptation, and I hope as well that, if worse comes to worse with one of his family members, he will care for them to the end, not even hinting they have a duty to spare him their troubles. I no less hope he will allow them the honor of caring for him until the end.

A DUTY TO CARE
Felicia Cohn and Joanne Lynn

Hardwig's notion of a "duty to die" is not foreign either to our medical culture or to society. Indeed, patients often say, "I just don't want to be a burden," and they mean it, emotionally, physically, and financially. Certainly, patients do turn down potentially beneficial treatment to avoid family impoverishment and hardship. In asking if we have a "duty to die," Hardwig raises an important question. His ruminations may have succeeded in "clarifying his own convictions," and he may even have helped some readers find personal answers.

However, despite its familiarity and Hardwig's earnest argument, the claim is no less demeaning to the elderly, frail, and sick in our society. That he is able to argue for a "duty to die" reveals much about our attitudes toward life, health care, and death. He builds his arguments on a number of troubling assumptions, neglects some important concepts, and ignores some problematic implications. First, Hardwig fails to consider the full impact of a "duty to die" on society and those who are actually dying in this country. Second, he takes for granted common fears and misperceptions about dying. Third, he misconstrues the debate in terms of rights and limited choices. Examination of Hardwig's claims reveals the issue is not that we **must** die, but **how** we die. The resolutions lie not in the obligation to die, but in the obligation to care for the dying.

The Impact of a "Duty to Die": The Price of Dying and Public Policy

A duty to die has some serious policy implications. Hardwig paints the issue too starkly, without considering the broad spectrum of circumstances in which people die. He neglects the impact on the meaning of life for the dying, particularly the elderly, and the relationship between a duty to die and other policy initiatives such as those related to health care reform and assisted suicide.

Hardwig's argument, driven by fears and misperceptions of dying, fails to find any meaning in the last phase of life. He goes so far as to suggest that even those who are not yet categorized as "dying" might incur a duty to die in order to avoid the tribulations associated with their eventual deaths. This reflects a societywide undervaluation of life's final journey. The elderly, the sick, and the dying have much to contribute and to gain; the end of life can be a very meaningful period. Articulating a duty to die would serve to reinforce the negative valuation surrounding aging and pervasive age-based biases.

Our society consistently rejects placing an explicit price on life, yet Hardwig's arguments violate the notion that life is priceless or sacred. As a matter of practicality, we do implicitly place values on continued existence, at least considering it as one good competing among others. Accepting an explicit duty to die, however, would unmask our euphemistic discussions, which are significant for maintaining our illusion that human life is priceless. The illusion is not a silly vanity; it conditions our attitudes and actions. We work hard to provide health care services to those in need, despite socioeconomic status. We do not let emergencies go unattended or allow individuals to die on the street. In accepting a duty to die, we would explicitly devalue life under certain circumstances and undermine an important cultural value. Society is more humane, kind, and protective when its members hold that every life is precious, even when nearing the end. As we die, we continue living. This period of life should not be stripped of its value and meaning. In the words of one "member of the generation that has outlived the conventional life span": "there's a growing number of oldsters still full of creaking vitality. Don't begrudge us respect."[1]

Individuals have not been called on previously to justify their continued existence. Accepting a duty to die means that the burden of proof will shift. Instead of an ongoing presumption in favor of life, any member of society could be required to make a case for his/her continued existence (at least to himself/herself and probably to his/her family). It is not clear how anyone could actually make that case. Moreover, such a radical shift in thinking about aging could have a profound impact in many arenas. What would it mean to our society if the general expectation were that some are obligated to die? And, would the adverse impact of that expectation fall disproportionately on specific persons or classes of persons? For example, how will a duty to die affect Social Security and Medicaid payments or the age of retirement? Will entitlement payments be denied to those who refuse to acquiesce, who refuse to give up living? Will the retirement age decrease so that people can enjoy some free time before ending their lives? Will supportive housing arrangements account for a particular rate of deliberately accelerated deaths? The government of China radically changed the structure of families when it prohibited families from having more than one child. Similarly, a duty to die could radically change how we live our lives and how we die. Rather than seeking ways to ensure meaningfulness until death, imposing a duty to die would evade any need to solve the problems associated with caring for those nearing death.

Drawing lines around this duty will also be difficult. A person can ordinarily decline chemotherapy but would be pressed to accept insulin, and can decline hospitalization near death but would be pressed to accept a blood test to diagnose the new onset of mild delirium. It seems few would support forgoing treatment that costs little, dramatically improves life prospects, and is rather ordinary in nature. However, definitions of little cost, improvement, and ordinary treatment are already controversial. How far should a duty to die go?

Directly implicated in this decision-making process is the debate over aid-in-dying. Hardwig's discussion fails to consider the nature and meaning of death and the current debate over assisted death. If we are to do away with ourselves prior to becoming burdensome, then we must have a means to death beyond the ordinary dying process. For some this could mean forgoing life-sustaining treatment; but for many, other forms of assistance will be necessary. Will a healthy person be expected to stop eating and drinking after recognizing the early signs of Alzheimer's disease? Will suicide become the most common cause of death? Must surrogate decision makers, not coincidentally the same family members who would bear the burdens and costs of care, lobby for lethal injections for their loved ones? Will each of us be expected to write an advance directive to authorize our killing in the event we are not able to take our own lives while we are still capable of doing so? The possibilities of and problems surrounding suicide, assisted suicide, and euthanasia complicate the question of whether a duty to die exists. Further, Hardwig does not account for the burden on survivors from even a "justifiable" suicide. It is reasonable to expect family and friends to be tormented by feelings of grief, inadequacy, and guilt following a family member's suicide. How are we to balance the burdens experienced by a family due to the premature and unnatural death of a loved one against the burdens imposed on a family in taking care of that elderly or dying loved one? Of what should our expectations consist: aid in dying or aid in living well while dying?

Even accepting that a duty to die is appropriate for some might alter the community's commitment to support those who are seriously disabled, especially those with immense service needs. Although not central to Hardwig's claims, it is troubling that his article includes drawings of restrained and sedated wheelchair-bound people. With regard to ordering our society, we must be careful of maudlin and misleading images. These images only feed the negative perceptions that become barriers to effective societal and policy changes. Hardwig admits that if better palliative and supportive care of the dying were available, a duty to die might become unnecessary or irrelevant. Instead of pressing for such reforms, he appears to accept that the system need not change. It is precisely the perceptions of a duty to die or the perceived need for assisted suicide that should incite us to improve the care available at the end of life. Public policy need not merely react to the culture in which it is developed, but can help shape that culture. New programs to provide care for dying persons and their families would not only address the array of problems most of us will face as we approach the end of life, but will also send a message: The final phase of life is valuable.

Common Fears and Misperceptions: Fear of Death
and the Technological Imperative

Hardwig's argument is symptomatic of the misperceptions about dying that pervade society. He buys into the expectations that society has come to have for health care: that aggressive medical care can conquer death and that families must bear the costs of these battles. In other words, he accepts society and health care as is. His response to the current context is a duty to avoid becoming a burden. The real burden, however, lies in this acceptance of the status quo. The goal need not be to eliminate those who become burdensome, but to decrease the burden. We should expect health care to enhance our final years, not to encumber or eliminate them.

Hardwig's arguments take for granted the current areas of focus and neglect in American medicine. While highlighting the use of technology to increase the length of life, we have ignored some of the implications of this usage. We have heralded longer life, but have not addressed the effects of a longer lifespan. We have not accepted that longer life does not mean extended youth. Nor have we recognized that while our health care system can extend life, it cannot address the needs associated with aging.

The health care system that has developed rests on and reinforces a societal and medical culture in which youth is prized and aging is treated as a disease to be cured. In the United States, the primary end of medicine appears to be the avoidance of death or the extension of life.[2] While we have become technologically capable of extending life, we cannot yet maintain youth and health. With longer life comes many health problems. Our health care system has yet to do much to address the complex needs of those who face these relatively new health problems, e.g., chronic heart disease, dementing illness, or a process of approaching death that may encompass many years. In pursuing extended life, quality of life is subsumed by quantity of life. In achieving extended life, the quality issues reemerge, revealing all too painfully the costs of extended life. A side effect of the great success of modern medicine is the advent of almost ubiquitous chronic illness. Most of us will be doomed to suffer as we die and will die slowly in the expensive hands of modern medical care.[3] The imperative, however, remains extending life, without regard to the needs of those living that extended life. These are the roots of a duty to die, as Hardwig explains: "A fairly common duty to die might turn out to be only the **dark side** of our life-prolonging medicine and the uses we choose to make of it."[4]

Only when mere continued existence is so highly and unconditionally prized could a duty to die evolve to the point of overwhelming a presumptive duty to live. Recognizing a duty to die indicates an acceptance of a dominant but narrow ethic: a technological imperative that requires cure despite the associated costs, both economic and human. Death is medicalized, transformed into a problem to be treated. The metaphor of war is pervasive in this context. We fight the enemy of disease with an arsenal of medicines. Death is the ultimate defeat. Fighting the war, especially a losing war, against disease does take a toll on the battlefield; when every day is a battle, a patient may prefer to surrender. Our health care system must learn to cater to the living of life even in the final phases rather than merely continuing existence and fighting to death. This qualitative difference would render a duty to die moot. Should dying become comfortable and meaningful, there would be no battles to fight and no need to hasten the process.

If dying is miserable and expensive, it is because we have allowed it to become that way. We must address the changes in how we die that have occurred over the last century. In 1900, we would likely have died at an age we now would consider young and would have experienced a relatively sudden death due to acute infection, childbirth, or rapidly progressing disease. Now we are more likely to die older, having lived with chronic illness for months or years. Our health care system has not responded to the technological advances of the last 40 years, retaining a system that is not prepared to handle the myriad needs of those approaching the end of life. Thus, we have come to fear the process of dying perhaps more so than death itself. The real duty then, lies not in doing away with ourselves when available resources become inadequate, but in facing those inadequacies. We must come to appreciate and facilitate the changes that occur in our bodies and minds throughout the course of life. We must change our response to dying.

Decisions and Choices: Rights Language and False Dichotomies

Hardwig chooses to frame the issue as a matter of dichotomous choices and decisions. The language he uses defines and constructs the questions and their answers. Rather than focus on the process of dying and the needs of those living through that process, the debate turns on decisions to be made in response to limited choices.

Hardwig's use of the term "duty" reflects the "rights" language[5] that has become so prevalent in health care issues. Rights, we learned in civics class, have correlative responsibilities. For example, if I have a right to drive, I also bear a responsibility to drive safely. Similarly, a right to die may entail a duty to die. That is, if I have a right to die, a just and proper claim to have my life end, then I might incur a responsibility to end that life appropriately. In a note, Hardwig disavows the "legalistic overtones" of this language. He notes that no law grounds this duty, but as a moral duty, the obligation is no less real. Whether legal or moral, reference to something as a duty entails obligation.

Death begins to look like a choice; i.e., one may choose to live OR choose to die. The circumstances of death become a matter of choice: to suffer with the disease health care professionals cannot treat or the patient will not treat OR to bring about an end to life. Even suffering becomes a choice: to seek comfort from suffering in the form of continued medical attention, possibly at the risk of impoverishing one's family, OR to suffer silently while maintaining the family inheritance. Decisions at the end of life take on a "me versus them" quality, which seems inapproriate or at least undesirable in the context of a family.

Without even considering the reciprocity possibly involved in family caregiving arrangements,[6] Hardwig trades on a particular notion of fairness that grows out of a Kantian sense of duty and a notion of family obligations. He appears to believe that such an obligation is a matter of universalizable law: that we should will all others in like situations to act similarly. Further, to expect one's family to bear the burden of one's preference for continued existence he believes renders family members as merely means to the dying person's end (i.e., living). Despite these explanations, Hardwig's analysis still appears to come down to a balance of burdens.[7] He even provides a list of considerations that must be weighed in considering the duty to die.[8] This is not a simple utilitarian calculus, but is utilitarian nonetheless. It is the "consequences for his loved ones" about which he appears to be most concerned.[9] A duty not to impose hardship on your family may exist. Certainly many patients express this feeling. But, as Hardwig admits, the duty to die is not incumbent upon those who are not wreaking havoc on their family's lives. The duty to die is contingent. When, exactly, does death become an obligation? For whom? Under what circumstances?

Matters of life and death are not best framed in terms of duties and choices. Death is neither a duty nor a choice so much as it is a fact. It may be more helpful to consider that we all reach a "time to die" rather than that we have a duty to die. It may be possible to retain some control over the timing and circumstances of death, e.g., via refusal of care, without acquiring an obligation to be dead. The mere existence of technology does not command its use. Additionally, we must distinguish between obligations to limit costs and burdens and an obligation to die. It is human choice that possesses the "dark side" Hardwig laments. The real choice to be had is not "to be or not to be," but how to use our resources appropriately as we "are." Further, this choice is not limited to any situation of "either/or": either to suffer and bankrupt or to die, either to treat or not to treat, either to cure or to comfort. The options include treating sometimes and not treating sometimes, curing as well as comforting. Even the amount of suffering we are forced to endure and the amount of money we must spend involve a range of choices. In fact, the very language used is a matter of choice. This is not merely a matter of semantics but of how we choose to care for those facing a situation we will all face eventually.

Conclusion

The issues Hardwig raises are and should be difficult. His arguments deserve harsh criticism, but this criticism has as much to do with our health care system and public attitudes as with Hardwig's philosophical musings. The concerns are not limited to health care professionals, policy makers, or the public. We will all face death one day, and very few of us will be fortunate enough to die suddenly, painlessly in our sleep after a rich 80 or 90 years of life. The inadequacies of the current health care system are not somebody else's problem. We will be stuck with the system we create—or the system we neglect. Hardwig's arguments and conclusions deserve attention, but we must work to ensure that criticism is constructive. We owe it to ourselves and our society's future to establish a duty to care.[10]

Notes

1. Argus J. Tresidder, "Longevity and Livability." *Newsweek* (March 2, 1998): 17.

2. Hardwig claims a duty to die is common in other, largely poor and technologically unsophisticated cultures. This may not be a duty so much as a reality. Without the ability or resources to extend life, individuals have choices only with regard to the attitudes they express toward dying. Death comes not as an imposition on a life too costly to continue, but as an acceptance, even a graceful acceptance, of mortality.

3. For a comprehensive description of the state of end-of-life care in the United States, see Institute of Medicine. *Approaching Death: Improving Care at the End of Life.* Washington, DC: National Academy Press, 1997.

4. J. Hardwig, "Is There a Duty to Die?" *Hastings Center Report* 27.2 (March–April 1997): 35. Emphasis added.

5. In discussing "rights language," we are drawing on Mary Ann Glendon's concept of "rights talk." She says:
"A tendency to frame nearly every social controversy in terms of a clash of rights (a woman's right to her own body vs. a fetus's right to life) impedes compromise, mutual understanding, and the discovery of common ground. A penchant for absolute formulations ("I have the right to do whatever I want with my property") promotes unrealistic expectations and ignores both social costs and the rights of others. . . . I have endeavored to demonstrate how our simplistic rights talk simultaneously reflects and distorts American culture. It captures our devotion to individualism and liberty, but omits our traditions of hospitality and care for the community."
Like Glendon, we seek the "indigenous languages of relationship and responsibility that could help to refine our language of rights" and to build on our tradition of care. It is in the recognition of responsibility within relationships that a duty to care lies. This duty extends beyond family as it involves creating a community context in which the final phase of life can be comfortable and meaningful. See Mary Ann Glendon. *Rights Talk: The Impoverishment of Political Discourse.* New York: The Free Press, 1991. xi–xii.

6. Hardwig does not account for arguments from family responsibility. Family members, particularly adult children, may believe they owe a sick parent care, as a reciprocal exchange for the care they received while growing up.

7. Hardwig, 38. "A duty to die is more likely when continuing to live will impose significant burdens—emotional burdens, extensive caregiving, destruction of life plans, and yes, financial hardship—on your family and loved ones. This is the fundamental insight underlying a duty to die."

8. Hardwig, 38–39. These factors to be considered include burdens imposed on family and loved ones, age, fullness of life, difficulties already faced by loved ones, previous contributions and sacrifices of loved ones, loss of mind and identity, and depleted savings.

9. Hardwig, 40. Hardwig later states: "Ending my life if my duty required might still be diffi-cult. But for me, a far greater horror would be dying alone or stealing the futures of my loved ones in order to buy a little more time for myself." Hardwig, 42. His expression of "greater horror" again suggests that he is pitting the value of his extended life against his family's future.

10. A duty to care involves more than a commitment by families to care for their elderly mem-bers. It would entail reform of our current health care system, including changes in health care financing mechanisms, service array, service sites, and eligible patient population. Hospice is a step in the right direction, but it serves only about 20 percent of those who die in the Medicare program. New programs have been proposed to address the complex array of needs individuals develop as they approach the end of life. See, for example, Joanne Lynn and Anne Wilkinson. "Quality End of Life Care: The Case for a MediCaring Demonstration." *A Good Dying: Shaping Health Care for the Last Months of Life*. Eds. Joan K. Harrold and Joanne Lynn. New York: Haworth Press, Inc., 1998. See also Joanne Lynn, Anne Wilkinson, Felicia Cohn, and Stanley Jones.."Capitated Risk-Bearing Managed Care Systems Could Improve End-of-Life Care." *Journal of the American Geriatrics Society* 46. (1996), 322–30.

SEEKING A RESPONSIBLE DEATH
Larry R. Churchill

Is there a duty to die? John Hardwig believes there is, and his essay makes a persuasive case for such a duty based on familial obligations, especially when coupled with the technological capacity to sustain a person over a long and expensive demise.[1] My aim here is to amplify and augment Hardwig's thesis. I agree that there is a duty to die, under certain circumstances, and I believe that this duty stems from both familial responsibilities and obligations to the preservation of the self. Since Hardwig has made a good case from familial obliga-tions, I will focus on the second rationale.

In undertaking this task I want to be clear that I speak only for myself. I am seeking to articulate a personally felt duty, not to instruct others. Still less do I want to suggest that there are implica-tions for health policy to be drawn from my argument, for example, consequences for health care financing or the setting of priorities about the use of scarce health resources. Current U.S. health policies systematically deny adequate health services to many of our most vulnerable citizens, and these denials are both cowardly and perverse. They are cowardly because they are cloaked in the rhetoric of "mar-ket forces"—for which no one takes responsibility;[2] they are perverse because they are often accompanied by moralizing about the "wor-thiness" of those who are ill served by the market-driven system, moralizing that tends to blame them for their ill health and lack of access.[3] In such an environment policy makers will be tempted to reduce moral arguments about a responsible death to actuarial tables of "winners" and "losers" and to turn a self-assumed and personal duty into a social obligation in the name of efficiency and cost control. I believe it would be a good thing if more persons felt a "duty to die," in the sense I will explicate, and also good if social customs and traditions were to support such a notion. But I am horrified by the thought that some such duty would become a part of health policy, complete with reimbursement schemes based on whether people fulfill this responsibility and penalties for those who are "irresponsible" and refuse to die in a timely and efficient fashion. My remarks here are about what I believe would be a good way to live one's life, including how to end that life, not arguments about what would be fair or just in terms of social policies for health care.

Although no policy implications should be drawn from my remarks, my thinking has been profoundly shaped by the increasing commercialization of health services, the negative impact of this commercialization on stable access to health care, and the potentially crippling cost of my care to those who will survive me. In more humane societies where stable and universal access to health services is a given, a duty to die would not present itself with the same urgency in terms of familial responsibilities, although arguments stemming from a concern for sustaining values that define the self might still be compelling.

Setting the Scene Realistically

As an ethics teacher I am frequently coaxing and cajoling learners to supply something from their moral sensibilities for me to work with—a case they find difficult, a value they strongly affirm, or an issue that perplexes or nags them. When the topic is care of the terminally ill, I often ask learners to fill out a death certificate on themselves, that is, to speculate on the timing, locations, and causes of their deaths. Most foresee their death occurring at an advanced old age, but with minimal loss of mental and physical capacity. Their deaths, as they envision them, most often occur at home and in their sleep, or in some exotic vacation site while engaged in vigorous athletic or sexual activity. And usually a significant percentage die on their birthdays. While a few foresee a premature death, these are almost always violent—automobile or skiing accidents; very few have died, in their imagination, from Alzheimer's disease. And to date no one has ventured to embrace a scenario that includes death by their own hand, undertaken as a responsibility to self and others.

These learners are largely medical and other health professional students, most of them in their mid-20s, and perhaps unable quite yet to imagine their own death. It is also likely that when asked to confront death all of us naturally seek reassuring scenes, rather than realistic ones. Yet the lack of realism is profound, for the deaths in store for most of us are not merely different from those forecast above, they are in diametrical opposition to them. Only these students' predictions about their age at death are likely to be accurate; the rest is fantasy. Death in the United States most often occurs in hospitals and nursing homes after years of declining vigor and with increasing personal expense, even for the well-insured.

Later in life we are more inclined to set the scene of our demise with greater clarity and less idealism and to reckon the financial and emotional costs, both to ourselves and to others. I cannot count on, and in truth have no reasonable expectation of experiencing, the death I want for myself. For me the death-of-my-desires occurs in my early 80s, while I am still finding new intellectual horizons to explore and new emotional layers to my life. Physically I am still intact, and while my death process may occur over months, or even years, it is not marked by pain, incontinence, physical or mental disability, or great expense. I have, in short, not become a burden to myself or others when I die. I still contribute, and my family and friends still see me as an interesting, engaging, and caring person. Moreover, the death-of-my-desires is one that is aesthetically pleasing and fitting for me as a unique individual. The end says something about the life as a whole, echoes the best of who I am, and in this sense is "appropriate." Perhaps I have just finished another essay for the Nelsons' latest volume in their ongoing *Reflective Bioethics* series or have published my first volume of haiku, now seen as one of the best vehicles for bioethics education. Or perhaps I have achieved a deeper level of affection with a member of my family. The possibilities are numerous and idiosyncratic, but the general desire for a death that shows something about one's life is very old and widely felt. Montaigne put this desire for an authentic death with characteristic clarity in his *Essays*: "[I]n the last scene, between death and ourselves, there is no more pretending; we must speak plain French, we must show what there is that is good and clean at the bottom of the pot."[4]

But who am I kidding? The chances are very good I will die with my last book or essay at least 10 years behind me, with only a part of my full mental abilities, and certainly only a fraction of my physical faculties in tow, in a hospital or a nursing home. I would be lucky, indeed, to get a quiet, dignified death on my 82nd birthday, surrounded by loving family and friends. I may well be overwhelmed by intractable suffering, loss of routine bodily functions, severe disability, progressive dementia, loss of financial means, and the absence of a nurturing convivial order to ease my pain and console my losses. Most horrifying, my dying process may also burden my progeny, drastically altering their life-prospects long after I am gone. This would wrong and harm them, but it would also damage my sense of self as I die. It would be a fate worse than death by my own hand.

Taking One's Own Life: Some Precedents

Once the scene is set realistically it becomes easier to pose the questions: "When would my death best occur?" "What will count as a good death for me?" Without the pretense that I can avoid death or that I am assured the death-of-my-desires, it becomes clear that I may have a choice. I am not, of course, assured of ever having a choice, for fate may conspire against me, taking away any choice in the matter. For example, I may fall dead from a massive heart attack some spring day while working in my yard or be crushed in an high-speed vehicular accident on Interstate 40, a victim of "road rage," an intoxicated driver, or just bad luck. Or I may suffer a stroke, lose consciousness or competence, and the burden of decisions will be passed to others. Yet I can also well imagine having a decision to make about when and how to die.

Decisions of this sort can be of two types: a decision to forgo further efforts at survival and a decision to actively end my life. The former has been long endorsed as a prerogative of persons to refuse treatment and as a prime example of patient self-determination. The latter has been almost uniformly criticized as morally unacceptable, stemming largely from religious arguments and from civic traditions that relied on religious doctrine. Although I find the term prejudicially laden with psychiatric overtones, this second form of a decision to die is essentially a question of "suicide", of whether and when to kill oneself. And despite the psychiatric bias, it is still preferable to most of the euphemisms, such a "self-deliverance" or "dropping the body," which fall prey to the same sort of wishful thinking as my students' imagined death scenarios. The act in question is one of killing oneself, of actively and deliberately taking one's own life. It is here that the argument should be focused.

"Suicide" as a term is only 300 years old, but the practice is surely as old as our species. In contrast to the Christian prohibition of this practice, accounts of ancient Greeks and Romans who took their own lives and are revered for their actions are numerous. The death of Socrates, although not technically a suicide in the contemporary sense, was a paradigm of a noble and self-chosen death. Socrates chose death over exile when his work in Athens was best served by his death and his continued life in exile could only diminish it. *Crito* is a locus classicus for a duty to die at the right time and for the right reasons. Central to the account of Socrates's death was his assertion that he had received a divine sign sanctioning his choice. This motif was central to some of the Stoic philosophers, especially Epictetus, who believed that Socrates had demonstrated the proper indifference toward death and that the question was not whether there is a proper time to remove oneself from life, but how to read the divine signals correctly.[5]

Interestingly, Jewish history is also marked by accounts of suicide that are viewed as fitting, or even praiseworthy. Abimelech, for example, the son of Gideon and an ironfisted military leader, dies during an attack on the city of Thebez. As Abimelech was attempting to burn down the fortified city, a Theban woman dropped a millstone on his head, crushing his skull. Sensing his predicament, Abimelech cried out to his armor-bearer, "Draw your sword and kill me, lest men say of me, 'A woman killed him.'" The armor-bearer obliged.[6] Saul, in a similar predicament and worried that the "uncircumcised" would kill him after "making sport" of him, made a similar request of his armor-bearer, who was less reliable, leaving Saul to do it himself. Finally, Samson, captured by the Philistines and being humiliated while standing between the central pillars of a building, was given divine strength to pull down the pillars, collapsing the building upon himself and the Philistines. As Arthur Droge and James Tabor have argued, the accounts of these "voluntary deaths" are remarkable not just for the absence of condemnation, but for the way in which the lives of these figures are in part redeemed by their manner of death.[7] This is especially the case for Saul and Samson. These accounts are, of course, also part of the Christian Bible, but occupy at best a dormant subtext to the dominant tradition, to which I now turn.

The Christian Prohibition and Its Critics

The official Christian doctrine about suicide is rooted not in the Gospels, or even in Scripture per se, but in the squabbles and power politics of the 5th century Church. Here the key figure is Augustine of Hippo and his efforts to defeat a view of martyrdom espoused by Donatus, one of Augustine's rival bishops of the early 5th century Church in northern Africa.[8] Followers of Donatus, called Donatists, sustained a tradition of voluntary martyrdom—actively embracing death in order to avoid apostasy, or even the violation of any law of God. Writing in a time of great persecution of Christians, and for a culture steeped in mind–body dualism, Augustine was faced with the problem of Donatists and other Christian zealots who engaged in reckless self-destructive acts. The aim was to escape the sins of this world and to attain, all the sooner, the bliss of the next. In this climate, and counter to these practices, Augustine argued that suicide is forbidden under the commandment against killing. He devised the theological trump card still being played: the belief that this present life is a providential test of spiritual worthiness. Killing oneself is, then, the avoidance of a divinely given responsibility, a refusal to complete the qualifying examination for the afterlife. Thomas Aquinas added two arguments to the Augustinian prohibition of suicide. He portrayed it as contrary to the charity one owes oneself and as a shirking of the duties owed to society, as well as a usurpation of the prerogatives of God.[9]

David Hume has provided the definitive refutation of the latter two arguments, which I will rehearse briefly before turning to the issue of how suicide bears upon duties to oneself. Hume draws upon Montesquieu in posing some of his arguments. For example, Montesquieu had argued that suicide does not disturb divine providence any more than other interventions into nature, such as changing the course of a river. Hume also borrowed from Stoic philosophers, especially the late Roman Stoics, who argued that if the disposal of human life were left exclusively to the Almighty, any act of avoiding death would be an infringement on divine sovereignty. In *Of Suicide*, Hume puts it this way: "If I turn aside a stone which is falling on my head I disturb the course of nature and invade the peculiar province of the Almighty by lengthening out my life beyond the period, which, by general laws of matter and motion, he had assigned to it."[10]

Moreover, Hume rightly observes that suicide could just as easily be seen as part of divine providence as opposed to it. "When I fall upon my sword, therefore, I receive my death equally from the hands of the deity, as if it had proceeded from a lion, a precipice, or a fever."[11] The argument, then, is something like this: Once I begin to interpret actions as expressions of divine will, there is no more reason to exclude suicide than to exclude diseases or accidents. If providence guides some causes, why not all? So Hume concluded, "Whenever pain or sorrow so far overcome my patience as to make me tired of life, I may conclude that I am recalled from my station, in the clearest and most express terms."[12]

Regarding the argument that there is a social obligation to continue living, even in circumstances burdensome to ourselves and others, Hume replied: "A man who retires from life does no harm to society; he only ceases to do good; which if it is an injury, is of the lowest kind . . . and where my life is a positive burden to society, my withdrawal from it is not only innocent but laudable."[13]

Of course, there may be other compelling arguments against suicide than those of Augustine and Thomas. Yet for those steeped in Calvinistic Christianity, such as Hume and myself, these arguments stood as the most important and compelling ones. Showing the flaws in their logic opens up possibilities for reconceiving my duty around life's end, a duty which is familial, but personal as well.

Honoring and Preserving the Self

I want to focus now on how a decision to end one's life can be a fulfillment of a duty to oneself, precisely the opposite of the Thomistic position that I have a duty of charity to myself never actively to end my own life.

The steps of thinking that lead to a duty to die begin with a realistic assessment of the human predicament. We are mortal beings, and death is not only the end result of life, but its telos—the aim or purpose for which we are headed biologically. It is our nature, a case elegantly made in a variety of places by Leon Kass.[14] Our natural rhythms are cyclical; we are structured to live and then to die. The question is not if, but when and how.

A second step involves clearing the space theologically. My life and death can be given meaning if I accept the Augustinian/Thomistic arguments that I will be called from my duties in life at precisely the right time and only in certain ways, namely, in ways that exclude taking my own life. Yet these arguments cannot sustain the desired conclusion, and indeed may support just the opposite conclusion. If God speaks to us, we may be required to end our lives as well as to preserve them. Here it is important to remember that Socrates and his Stoic admirers, as well as Samson, were called to take their lives by divine instruction. The overall lesson is that divine commands, even those mediated through centuries of tradition, form an equivocal basis for action, a double-edged argument about suicide, rather than a clean case against it.

But divine instruction is only a part of the tradition of a good death in the examples discussed here. The more relevant feature is that death is, ironically, undertaken as an avenue of self-preservation, a way of preserving and honoring what is distinctive about one's own life or, at a minimum, a way to avoid a death that is demeaning, humiliating, or diminishes the basic values one has tried to embody. If our distinctiveness as individual people involves how we live and what we make of our lives, if living is more than biological inertia and unthinking habituation, the embodiment of these core values must count heavily in any reckoning of a "good" death. While few late 20th century Americans would interpret a catastrophic death as one at the hands of a woman, or by the "uncircumcised," tens of thousands of Americans have enough fear of a demeaning or humiliating death through technological extensions of a low-level "quality of life" that they have signed living wills and arranged for durable powers of attorney for health decisions. Israelite chieftains and Roman generals fell on their swords; many Americans fall back on their doctors, relatives, and lawyers to ensure that their deaths will not diminish the values they have lived by, seeking thereby to preserve in their deaths the selves they have been. But of course the success of this advance directive strategy for preserving the self presupposes a clear occasion on which life supports can be withdrawn or forgone, allowing death to ensue. I would be lucky, indeed, if this were the case for me. Such a scenario would qualify as a second best in my desirable-death scenarios, second to dying peacefully at home with all my faculties at my 82nd birthday party.

Montaigne, with debts to both Solon and Ovid, entitled one of his *Essays* "That Our Happiness Must Not Be Judged Until After Our Death."[15] The phenomenon he wanted to signal through this title is the human desire to die at the right time, in the right way, and for the right reasons and the precariousness of achieving such a death. In my sanguine moments I know this is unlikely to occur. I also know that I can tolerate many kinds of death that might tarnish my sense of self, but that some are unspeakably horrible because they would repudiate everything I believe my life is about. Some would cause me to say (if still able to speak), along with Montaigne, "I have lived longer than I should."[16]

Perhaps it is excessive vanity that causes me to think that my death should bear the weight of exhibiting the self. Yet I don't want it to bear the revelatory burden suggested by Kubler-Ross's portrayal of good dying as "the final stage of growth."[17] I simply want a death that is "mine," in some authentic sense. Although I hope to learn from my dying, I have no desire for a new self, kindled in the dying experience, and I resist strongly the idea that my dying will reveal to me that it is all right to have others be excessively burdened by my death because they will then be enabled to exercise compassion and sacrifice, and that I will learn the virtues of dependence. I do not fear dependence per se, but I do fear a level of dependence that is devoid of reciprocity and mutuality.

It is not vanity but a proper self-respect (and perhaps a touchy sense of pride) that seeks values roughly commensurate with my life to be displayed through my death. In this sense, my death can and should ideally be a vehicle for my self, just as I am concerned that other facets of my life carry this weight. Here again, Montaigne has an apt phrase: "The advantage of living is not measured by length, but by use: some men have lived long and lived little; attend to it while you are in it. It lies in your will, not in the number of years, for you to have lived enough."[18]

I do not pretend that achieving this preservation of self through taking my own life would be easy. I do not assume it would be simple for my family and friends to fully understand this, although I do not find these conversations any more difficult than others that concern the shape, texture, and means to embody deeply held values. If Montaigne is right and it lies in my will, I may not possess the will, or the courage, if given the occasion, to carry though with what I have embraced here. Or at some future date I may well decide that I was wrong, decades ago, when I wrote this. New stages of life teach new lessons, and if I am lucky enough to live into my 70s or 80s, I may see a different wisdom. For now, I see seeking a responsible ending as not only a duty to family, but a duty to myself, a final way of attempting to say and show what there is "at the bottom of the pot."

Notes

1. John Hardwig. "Is There A Duty to Die?" *Hastings Center Report* 27.2 (1997): 34–42.

2. See Larry R. Churchill. *Rationing Health Care in America-Notre Dame Press*, IN: U of Notre Dame P, 1987. 14–15.

3. See Dan Beauchamp. "Public Health as Social Justice." *Inquiry* 13 (1976): 4–6.

4. Michel de Montaigne. *The Complete Essays of Montaigne*, trans. Donald M. Frame. Stanford, CA: Stanford U P, 1965. 55.

5. Epictetus. *The Handbook of Epictetus*, trans. Nicholas White. Indianapolis: Hackett Publishing, 1983.

6. Accounts of the deaths of Abimelech, Saul, and Samson are taken from *The Oxford Annotated Bible*, eds. Herbert G. May and Bruce M. Metzger. New York: Oxford U P, 1965. Abimelech's death is recorded in Judges 9:50–57, Saul's in I Samuel 31:2–5, and Samson's in Judges 16:23–31.

7. Arthur J. Droge and James D. Tabor. *A Noble Death: Suicide and Martyrdom Among Christians and Jews in Antiquity*. New York: Harper Collins, 1992., 59. Droge and Tabor prefer the term "voluntary death" to avoid the bias of "suicide."

8. Augustine. *Concerning the City of God Against the Pagans*, trans. Henry Bettenson. New York: Penguin Books, 1984. 31–41. See also the excellent discussion of Augustine's views in Droge and Tabor.

9. Thomas Aquinas. *Summa Theologica*, 2nd part, 2nd number, question 64, article 5.

10. David Hume. "Of Suicide." *David Hume: Essays, Moral, Political and Literary*, rev. ed., ed. Eugene F. Miller. Indianapolis: Liberty Classics, 1985, 583.

11. Ibid., 584.

12. Ibid., 585.

13. Ibid., 586–87.

14. See, for example, Kass's "Mortality and Morality: The Virtues of Finitude" in *Toward a More Natural Science*. New York: Free Press, 1985. 299–317. While I espouse Kass's celebration of human finitude, I do not suggest that he would embrace my views on taking one's own life.

15. Montaigne, 54–55.

16. Ibid., 55.

17. Elisabeth Kubler-Ross. *Death: The Final Stage of Growth*. Englewood Cliffs, NJ: Prentice-Hall, 1975.

18. Montaigne, 67.

Dying Responsibly

Reflections on These Commentaries

"A responsible death"—that's it, precisely. Churchill's phrase nicely captures the central point. One can live responsibly or irresponsibly. Accordingly, one can age responsibly or irresponsibly; one can respond to illness, disability, debility, or harbingers of dementia responsibly or irresponsibly. And one can die responsibly or irresponsibly.

Churchill helpfully distinguishes responsibilities to others from responsibilities to self and reminds us that we may need to end our lives in order to remain true to ourselves. I will return briefly to responsibilities to self. But my focus here will be on responsibilities to others. Much more still needs to be said about a death that is responsible to others.

It is irresponsible and wrong to make decisions that ignore the needs, values, and interests of others. We should not, then, get diverted by semantics or the metaethics of "duty" at the very beginning of a critically important moral discussion. Callahan, and Cohn and Lynn insist that to claim someone has a duty to die implies—by virtue of the mere logic of "duty"—that someone else has a *right* that this person die. That's just not true.[1] I do not think we should cede the word "duty" to a rights-based ethics. But even more, I do not think we should get sidetracked into a discussion of the word. If "duty" is a problem, we can just as well begin, at least, by considering a responsible death.

There is now a vast literature about a good death, a literature in which the idea of a responsible death is rarely, if ever, mentioned. Of course, there is much more to a good death than dying responsibly.

But surely an irresponsible death cannot be called a good death, regardless of how peaceful and comfortable it may have been for the one who died. Similarly, an irresponsible way of coping with chronic illness, debility, or dementia cannot be called a good adjustment, no matter how pleased the patient and her physician may be with the results.

Autonomy and Responsibility

All this seems so obvious. And yet, patient responsibility is not a common theme in bioethics. We have seen a 30-year effort on the part of virtually all bioethicists, and many doctors and nurses, to empower patients to make decisions about their medical treatment. That's the patient autonomy movement. It still dominates bioethics, especially at the bedside. But with freedom comes responsibility—when you have or are given power to make choices that will affect the lives of others, you bear responsibility. Unavoidably so. That's just a fact of life.

Yet bioethics is almost completely silent about the responsibilities of autonomous patients. Similarly, Callahan, Cohn and Lynn, and Hentoff all have nothing to say in their essays about the responsibilities of autonomous patients. They, together with most bioethicists, implicitly invite us to ignore our responsibilities by talking as if the central question about medical treatment is simply what a patient wants. As if there could be freedom without responsibilities. As if freedom meant simply the opportunity to choose whatever you want for yourself. Those who try to live responsibly know that often the most important question is not what you want.

Bioethicists must learn to recognize that death is often quite literally "a death in the family." As such, it is usually a critical event for everyone involved. The circumstances of death are often more important and significant to the patient's family and close friends than to the patient herself. The same is true for chronic illness, debility, or dementia. Indeed, a serious illness or death is often much more difficult for the rest of the family than for the one who is ill or dies. We must not lose sight of these facts. We must not pretend that only the patient's interests are at stake in the medical response to illness and impending death. For the patient may well have less at stake in medical treatment decisions than her loved ones.

This volume works toward a family-centered bioethics. A bioethics that is family-centered would begin with an honest recognition that many treatment decisions have a major impact on the lives of family and loved ones. Our responsibilities to others when we are seriously ill or dying may well reach farther than responsibilities to those who are close to us. But surely, at a minimum, our responsibilities encompass ongoing watchful concern for the well-being of our loved ones. The decisions we make when we are seriously ill and dying will often dramatically alter the rest of their lives.

Autonomy is a central value. But from a family-centered perspective, this means that we must respect and promote the autonomy of *all* whose lives are affected, not only the autonomy of the one family member who happens to be sick. The ethics of family life will not condone arrangements that promote and support the autonomy of one family member while obliterating the autonomy of the rest. Our present bioethics of patient autonomy routinely does precisely that. If we employ an ethics of patient autonomy, I will have to use my autonomy when I am ill to protect and promote the autonomy and well-being of my loved ones, not just to further my own.

In my time of need, this may be very difficult to do. Yet in light of the devastating impact that serious illness and death can have on an entire family, we might well expect the responsibilities of the chronically ill or dying to be extensive, weighty, and perhaps severe. And I may be seriously ill, debilitated, or struggling with the prospect of my death. I may not be in very good shape to bear such heavy responsibilities.

If the responsibilities that come with patient autonomy seem too much to bear or too much to ask, there is another option: "Roll back the whole patient autonomy movement. It was a bad ethical mistake. It looked like a good idea at first, but only because we overlooked the responsibilities that come with autonomy. We can't ask sick, debilitated, and dying people to bear those kinds of responsibilities. Patient autonomy is fine for minor illnesses and for treatments that do not significantly affect the lives of others. It may be fine for those who are all alone, without family or close friends. But since major medical decisions almost always have important implications for the patient's families and loved ones, we should develop a bioethics that would lift the burdens of autonomy from patients."

The idea that some are not capable of being responsible has governed our approach to children, those with serious mental illnesses, and the demented. Analogously, perhaps those who are ill are not capable of choosing responsibly. Perhaps serious illness has a way of blinding us to the interests of others or making us incapable of choosing in light of them. And even if sick people are *capable* of choosing responsibly, perhaps we should not ask them to do so. They are in the throes of the crisis of failing health and often of impending death, as well. If the responsibilities that come with freedom are just too weighty, there is only one way to solve that problem—we can remove the responsibilities only by removing the freedom.[2]

But I contend that this option is insulting. It is insulting to a competent, adult patient to speak to her or of her as if she had no responsibilities to consider in making treatment decisions—it is to imply that she is morally incompetent or so compromised by her illness that we should not ask her to be responsible. Human dignity does not rest *solely* on the ability to choose responsibly, as Callahan would have me say. But if one is competent, it is plainly an assault on her dignity to treat her as if she had no responsibilities or were unable to respond appropriately to them.

Callahan's rhetoric sometimes carries him perilously close to implying that sick and dying people have no responsibilities to others. But I assume that Callahan, Cohn and Lynn, and Hentoff would all agree with me so far. None of them, I think, would contend that autonomous patients somehow have no responsibilities. Nor would they advocate abandoning patient autonomy, due to the weight of responsibilities autonomy brings with it. So I presume the disagreements among us would come over issues of how far this responsibility can reach. What might be involved in a responsible death?

Of course, responsibility runs both ways within a family. The young and healthy have responsibilities to the old, the sick, and the dying. Most families meet those responsibilities very well. Still, all resources of a family should not be directed toward one member, except for a short period of time. But what if I can be sustained in my illness only by a total dedication of their resources? What then?

MEDICAL VITALISM AS A FAMILY VALUE

Some might claim that there are no limits to what families ought to do to prolong the life or promote the health of a member of their family. Callahan quotes Frost's famous line: "Home is where, when you have to go there, they have to take you in." That is effective rhetoric until we ask what it really means. If you go home, many families will be unable to turn you away, especially if you are seriously ill.

Your presence will be compelling—it will force family members and loved ones to do all sorts of things for you. They will often feel they simply have no other choice. As the poet says, they have to take you in.

Perhaps having to take you in is not only psychologically compelling, but also morally justified. There are no moral limits to what families must do to respond to illness. They must bear whatever burdens are necessary to support the well-being of the sick, the debilitated, or the dying.

This view turns out to be a close cousin of medical vitalism, the belief that prolonging life is the highest value. Indeed, longer life and better health *must* be the ultimate values in order to justify the demand that *all* other goals and values of the family be sacrificed to prolong the life of a family member. This form of medical vitalism differs from the older version only in requiring that more life be desired by the one facing death.

Moreover, when there is uncertainty about whether an incompetent patient would want to continue to live as she now is, most bioethicists counsel us to presume that she would. Thus, longer life is the ultimate value if only it is desired or can be presumed to be desired. At the bedside, longer life is taken to be the highest value unless it has been explicitly revoked by the patient.

Both the new and the older versions of medical vitalism are to be rejected. Thanks in no small part to the work of Callahan and Lynn, we are beginning to recognize that we need to reform our medicine and our health care system so that they are no longer governed by an unlimited fight against death. Prolonging life as long as it is desired is not a good ultimate value around which to orient a health care system. Other goals for health care are simply more important. But if medical vitalism is not an appropriate pole star for a health care system, it is certainly even worse as a highest value for a family.

But ironically, even as we talk about reforming our medicine away from a commitment to medical vitalism, every day in practice we conscript families to live under its banner. For we force them to subordinate all other values and goals to prolonging life and promoting health, provided only that the patient has not explicitly denied that she wants her life prolonged. When we heroically rescue chronically ill patients from acute episodes and then discharge them back home—where they have to take you in—we often effectively reduce families to "patient-support systems" and nothing more. For all their resources—time, energy, emotional support, caring, money—will be required to deal with the consequences of our medical effort to prolong the life of the patient.

I do not see how it can be morally cogent to argue that our health care system should not be committed to prolonging life at whatever cost while simultaneously requiring families to prolong life at whatever cost to them. But if my family is not to be required to live out a medical vitalism, there are limits to what they can legitimately be asked to do to support and sustain me.[3] They must not sacrifice all other values on the altar of my medical care or even my desire to avoid death. I cannot responsibly ask them to do so.

Look at it another way. Consider the following question:

Q: The rest of my family should do everything they can to:
    a. help me achieve my career goals
    b. help me achieve my educational objectives
    c. help me get closer to God
    d. help me prolong my life and promote my health
    e. help me find real love and deep friendships
    f. none of the above

I think the correct answer to this question is "f"—none of the above. Not everything they can, at least not for more than a very limited period of time. All members of a family should be willing to make sacrifices to help each other achieve these goals. But I am not the center of my family; all the rest should not subordinate their lives to my goals. Why should my desire to live longer trump all of their goals and values? Besides, I submit that "d" is not the correct answer—of the values listed above, a longer life is not the preeminent value, the moral trump to which all other values must always be subordinated.

So there are limits. Except for short periods of time, it would be *wrong* for any member of my family to devote all her energy or other resources to my care. For that would leave no resources for the care of herself, her other loved ones, or the rest of the family, to say nothing of her responsibilities beyond the family. To ask my family to devote all their resources to my care or to put them in a position in which they feel they have to do so is often irresponsible.

Of course, there are any number of things I can do which might effectively force my family to do more than they can rightly be asked to do. But if I do these things, I have behaved irresponsibly. I have wronged them. They may have no recourse and no means to protect themselves. They simply have to take me in. So I may well be able to get away with it. But if I do, I would have wronged them and would need forgiveness for what I have done to them.

There is, then, a higher morality: of all places, home is where you must not go if going there would ruin the lives of everyone else there or force them to become mere auxiliaries to your projects, including your desire to live longer. One elderly woman said to a group of other seniors, "Don't ever, *ever* say to your children, 'Promise me you won't ever put me in a nursing home.' And if you've already said that, go to your children, take it back, and apologize for having said it." Here is a morality much more sensitive to what "going home" can mean to your loved ones.

So we come again to the question: What if it seems that I have to go home because I cannot live independently and there is no other place for me to go? What if I can be sustained in my illness only by a near total dedication of my family's resources? What then? Sometimes, I still must not go home. Not even then. These are the situations in which I believe that I may well have a responsibility to end my life.

HOW FAR CAN RESPONSIBILITIES TO LOVED ONES REACH?

The idea that there is a fairly common duty to die is a bitter pill to swallow. Perhaps, then, it would be worth asking whether smaller doses of this medicine would be more palatable. Perhaps seriously ill or debilitated people have responsibilities, but they do not go that far. How far can the responsibilities of the chronically ill, the aged, and the dying extend?

Clearly, a responsible death involves much, much more than simply declining medical treatments or even ending your own life. Indeed, that might not even be the hardest part of responsibly facing chronic illness or the end of your life. For example, moving out of your home or spending years in a nursing home may be much more difficult than ending your life. Nevertheless, bioethics has been focused almost exclusively on the ethics of treatment decisions and suicide. So that seems an appropriate place to center the present discussion of a responsible death. But we must remember that this focus omits other equally important dimensions of a responsible death.[4]

Consider, then, the responsible acceptance or refusal of medical treatment. Most bioethicists talk as if these decisions should be governed solely by what the patient wants. But that's to talk as if decisions about medical treatment brought no responsibilities with them. So, can there be a responsibility to refuse medical treatment? Even if that treatment is life-prolonging? Even if one wants that treatment for oneself?

> A 62-year-old teacher has a condition that might well progress to the point at which a bone marrow transplant would be the only treatment that could save his life. But that treatment is not covered by his insurance and the cost of it would obliterate his family's savings, leaving his wife destitute. She is retired, also in her 60s, and would not be able to recoup those savings. Their children are struggling financially and in no position to pay for the transplant. This couple has talked it over and decided together that he will not accept a bone marrow transplant. To accept it, he believes, would be an irresponsible way to respond to his illness. If it comes to that, he will die instead. When asked whether he would accept the transplant if he were single and childless, he responds without a moment's hesitation: "Sure! Why not?"

This is not an uncommon story. It happens all the time. The teacher's main difficulty is not one of deciding what he wants for himself. That part is easy—he wants to live. Nor is the central issue whether the pain and disability caused by the treatment itself is too great to go through in order to live—he would gladly undergo the necessary treatment. The central issue he faces is whether he can responsibly choose the treatment he wants for himself. He and his wife have concluded that he cannot.

Callahan, Cohn and Lynn, and Hentoff are all appalled at the idea that one might have a responsibility to take one's own life. It is a troubling idea. But one wonders what they would say about the decisions this man—this couple—face. Would they admit that one can have a responsibility to decline life-prolonging treatment? If not, perhaps they believe, after all, that there can be no such thing as an irresponsible death.

I cannot say for sure whether this teacher has a responsibility to decline this life-saving treatment because I don't know enough about his wife, their marriage, and their family life. The responsibilities of the seriously ill to their loved ones are very contextual.[5] But I think this couple's decision is probably the right one—it may well be irresponsible for him to accept the transplant. In any case, it would clearly be irresponsible for him to accept the transplant simply on the grounds that "I want to live." Of course he wants to live. But that is not a good enough reason for someone in a situation like his. Not if he would approach his illness and death responsibly.

What medical treatments can there be a responsibility to decline? Surely not just single, high-tech, very expensive interventions like a bone marrow transplant. For a series of smaller expenses or a prolonged period of chronic illness may, quite predictably, be more draining on loved ones than a large, one-time expense. The line between treatments that may be responsibly accepted and those that may not be does not fall between expensive, high-tech and inexpensive, simple treatments. There can be a responsibility to decline simple, inexpensive treatments, too.

What about medically supplied food and water? Most physicians and bioethicists agree that patients have the right to refuse *all* medical treatments, including medically supplied food and water . . . at least for self-interested reasons. And in practice, artificial nutrition and hydration are now commonly withdrawn when we acknowledge that they serve only to prolong the dying process or a life that is of unacceptably poor quality. Dr. Lynn has been at the forefront of the movement to establish the right of patients to refuse even this sort of treatment.[6]

But what if *others* would be better off if the disease process did not take so long to end the patient's life? Can there be a *responsibility* to decline even medically supplied food and water? If not, why cannot the responsibilities involved in making medical treatment decisions reach that far? I believe there are situations in which it would clearly be irresponsible and wrong for me to accept artificial nutrition and hydration.

I believe there can be a responsibility to decline life-prolonging or health-enhancing medical treatments. I believe it is fairly common. If one declined *all* life-prolonging medical treatments, a responsible death would only rarely have to involve suicide. If my critics can admit that there can be a responsibility to decline all life-prolonging medical treatments, they can go with me perhaps 90 percent of the way to my conclusion. I will almost always be able to avoid being a morally unjustifiable burden on my loved ones if I carefully and judiciously refuse medical treatments.

Almost always, but not always:

1. There are times when death by disease treated only by palliative care will be a much worse death—for me, for my loved ones, or

for all of us—than some of the alternative ways of dying. We can medicate the physical pain, but that does not relieve the suffering of the patient and also the family. We must candidly acknowledge that there are such cases. Lynn and Cohn argue we must reform our health care system to reduce the number of cases in which a horrible death would result from refusing treatment. I certainly agree. Still, there remain important questions about whether ethics truly mandates a much worse death when a better death (by suicide) is available. Is there something about death at one's own hand that makes it morally unjustifiable, even when that prohibition dooms me and my loved ones to a much worse end of my life? Callahan clearly thinks there is.[7] I am not convinced.

2. There are also cases in which declining medical treatments is not sufficient because none is required to prolong my life, which is nevertheless taking a horrible toll on my loved ones. Alzheimer's disease in someone who is otherwise in splendid health comes to mind as one possible example.

For these two kinds of cases, I believe there can be a responsibility to end one's life. Others may not be able to accept the idea that one ever has a responsibility to take one's own life. (Not *ever*?) But there may yet be substantial agreement. If we can agree that there can be a strong responsibility to decline medical treatments, then we have broad and important moral agreement. The remaining disagreement about suicide, although sometimes critically important, would come into play in relatively few cases.

THE SOCIAL SETTING AND A DUTY TO DIE

The responsibilities of a seriously ill person to her loved ones are contextual—they depend on many nuances and details of the family in which she has lived. But a person's responsibilities also depend on her social context. Consequently, a sick or dying person's responsibilities will depend on the health care system, including the insurance system, and on the ways in which families are required to bear or are sheltered from the burdens of chronic illness, debility, dementia, or a protracted dying process in their family.

Let us return to the example of the teacher in need of a bone marrow transplant. Perhaps the most common response to this story is that the teacher and his wife shouldn't have to be in this situation: "That's terrible! The teacher's health insurance company should pay for the transplant! And if it refuses, it should be forced to pay for one." That's quick and easy. It's emotionally appealing. But it may or may not be true. We live in a social context that mandates cost containment in health care. Employers and the government either cannot or will not continue to pay more and more for health care. In such a context, if it becomes more expensive to insure people, the result will be that fewer people will have health insurance of any kind. Given all this, paying for bone marrow transplants involves very complex trade-offs. Perhaps the teacher's health care plan does more good by paying for something else instead of bone marrow transplants, even if some people will die for lack of a transplant.

But the suspicion that the insurance company should pay will not be so easily quieted: "If the insurance company or health care plan were not so bent on generating profits for its shareholders, it could afford to pay for bone marrow transplants!" Or, "If the chief executive officers of the HMO were not paid such outrageous salaries, the plan could easily afford to pay for the transplant!" Or yet, "If employers are unwilling to pay for health care plans that cover the cost of *all* needed treatments, the government should step in and provide treatment for those who need it!"

Again, these claims seem obvious and morally right-headed. But the assumptions embodied in them may or may not be true. The view that profits are the problem goes against the capitalist philosophy that governs our whole society. We believe in capitalism enough to impose it on the rest of the world. Our food, housing, clothing, and transportation are all brought to us by for-profit corporations. Increasingly, our child care, utilities, prisons, and education are also provided by for-profit organizations. Why not our health care, too?

Most of us deeply believe that we get better value for our money from for-profit organizations than we would from non-profit corporations or the government, despite the profit motive and the profits generated. To believe otherwise is to take a huge step toward embracing socialism. Is health care really an exception? If so, why? Not because health care is a necessity that some people can ill afford—food, clothing, and shelter are all provided primarily on a for-profit basis.

We in the United States also live in an economic context in which executives of corporations are very handsomely rewarded. The current view in our country (though not so much in Europe or Asia) is that a good CEO is extremely valuable, well worth millions of dollars per year in compensation. We seem to believe that we get more and better goods and services at a cheaper price if we pay CEOs millions per year than if we find someone who will do the job for much less. In a context in which the CEO of one chain of clothing stores recently earned $44 million for one year, can we really expect executives in the much more complex and controversial world of health care not to receive roughly similar compensation packages?

Maybe it's true that "the government" should step in and pay for this man's bone marrow transplant. Perhaps the government should provide care (not just medical treatments!) for everyone who cannot take care of themselves. If the government would pay for this kind of care, a duty to die would be extremely rare, not relatively common, as I believe it is today.

But it's also true that we live in a social context defined by the taxpayer revolt. Only the most courageous (or foolhardy) of politicians dares to run on a platform of higher taxes to pay for, say, better education or more health care. Those who do are usually defeated. In this context, it may be politically impossible for any government agency to pay for all the health care we need. But more importantly, it may not even be true that the government should pay for more health care. Other needs—education, environmental protection, revitalizing our cities, better rehabilitation efforts for juvenile first offenders—may well be more important.

(Most of us must confess that we are part of the taxpayer revolt. I sometimes ask audiences: How many feel that your taxes are far too low? Usually only one or two hands go up. This is the context in which our government must decide how much funding to devote to health care. Interestingly, even health care providers apparently would not vote to tax themselves to provide needed health care for everyone. At least, when I ask audiences composed of health care professionals who would support increased taxes for themselves for this purpose, very few raise their hands.)

Perhaps unfavorable publicity or a court of law could force the health care plan to pay for the teacher's bone marrow transplant, whether or not it should. Probably not, though. This man is not a very compelling "poster child," and there may be no lawyer willing to take his case on a contingency basis. Obviously, it will not help his family's financial situation if they spend thousands of dollars trying to force the health care plan to pay.

Now, it is critical to notice one common feature of all these hypothetical responses to the teacher's moral dilemma. They all say that he should not have to face this moral dilemma because his situation should be different than it is. That may or may not be true. *But even if it is true*, that is really irrelevant to this couple's dilemma. It is simply not helpful to point out that someone else should pay for the transplant. Because no one will do so. This couple's decision must be made in their actual moral context, not in some better world in which that context would be different.

It would be grossly irresponsible for the teacher to accept the transplant on the grounds that the government or his health care plan should pay for it. For he knows that in fact neither will do so. Refusing the only medical treatment that could save his life may then be the only responsible course for him to take.

It is also largely irrelevant to his moral context that this teacher has always supported higher taxes for health care and for a much stronger social safety net. Unfortunately for him, his vision is not the one that has shaped his moral context. A person's moral context— and hence her *individual* responsibilities—is shaped not only by her own choices, but also by large-scale public choices and also by literally millions of individual choices that other people make.

Put more generally, the point is this: Any society must decide whether to bear the burdens of the unfortunate collectively or individually. Insurance (public or private), Social Security and retirement funds (public or private), and welfare plans are all devices that allow us to bear responsibility collectively. Under a system of collective responsibility, those who are fortunate enough not to have family members who become seriously ill or who cannot care for themselves subsidize those who are not so lucky, and we all insure ourselves against having huge burdens fall upon us or our loved ones.

Accordingly, we could decide to tax ourselves to provide collectively for the needs—not just the health care!—of people who can't care for themselves. That's what Canada is trying to do. When I talked about a duty to die in Canada, I was told that no one in Canada is impoverished by an illness in their family. By contrast, in the United States tens of thousands of families are impoverished every year by medical treatment decisions.[8]

But the emphasis in the United States today is on individual responsibility. The popular idea in this country is that each person should be responsible for herself and families should take care of their own, without looking to the rest of us for much help. This approach may well reduce our taxes. But that is not the end of the matter. A social decision not to bear responsibility collectively does not mean that responsibilities simply evaporate. Rather, it increases our individual responsibilities, sometimes dramatically. If we choose not to provide collectively for those in need, we must protect and provide for our loved ones individually.

As we reshape our social context, we also redefine our personal responsibilities. The renewed emphasis on individual responsibility brings with it the consequence that many more Americans will face a duty to die. Each of us must live and die in the social context we create together: Either we will bear responsibilities collectively or we will have to face them individually—often in terms of personal caregiving, sometimes in the sacrifice of health, and even—if I am correct—in decisions to lay down our own life.[9]

The Ethics of Contexts and Ethics within a Context

Clearly, some contexts are more morally justifiable than others. The attempt to discover which contexts are more justifiable—the ethics of contexts—is very important. It is a central part of ethics and of bioethics. In addition, bioethicists and others should advocate for the creation of a more justifiable moral context. That, too, is very important. Pointing out that our medicine or health care system should be reformed is part of the ethics of contexts. The claim that someone should pay for bone marrow transplants is also part of the ethics of contexts.

But the story of the teacher and his wife makes it clear that we must do more than attempt to discern and advocate for better moral contexts. Ethics within the present context is just as critical. So we must also try to figure out what is the right thing to do, *given* the context in which we actually do live, including the way it is likely to evolve. For our actual moral choices must be shaped by our actual social and personal contexts.

My essay on the duty to die is an essay about one facet of a responsible death in our present social context. I believe it will remain in effect until the reforms promoted by bioethicists and others are in place.

Cohn and Lynn maintain that instead of accepting a duty to die, we should reform our medicine and our health care system. I agree with every single reform they advocate. If these reforms came about, they would substantially reduce the number of people who have a duty to die. But, in contrast with Cohn and Lynn's view, I maintain that we must recognize that there is a duty to die in our present social context and there will be one at least until the reforms they advocate are realized.

Cohn and Lynn also think that admitting a duty to die is politically unwise—it will tempt insurers to scale back payment for the care of seriously ill and dying patients. They would be unjustified in doing so.[10] But if we are talking political strategy, I would propose another: admit that thousands of Americans now confront a responsibility to end their lives, that even larger numbers will probably face a duty to die in the near future, and that this situation can be alleviated only by basic reforms in our health care system.

If we are uncomfortable with a duty to die, we can reform our health care and welfare systems to minimize it. Conservative politicians and advocates of "family values" might well have second thoughts about their insistence on individual and family responsibility if confronted with the responsibility to die that their positions imply for many Americans.

I myself am a strong believer in a system of collective responsibility. This belief is strengthened by my reflections on the weighty responsibilities that must be borne by unlucky individuals and their unfortunate families if a system of collective responsibility is not in place. I would happily pay much higher taxes to establish a genuine safety net for all Americans. If the social context I advocate were in place, the individual responsibilities of the chronically ill, the debilitated, and the dying would be much lighter. A responsibility to end your life would be rare.

But all these personal convictions are largely irrelevant to my views about a duty to die for at least three reasons: (1) These views all amount to convictions that our social context should be different then it is. We do not live in the world I advocate. (2) Realistically, I must admit that the reforms I advocate are not likely to be enacted any time soon. As I have said, we are moving in just the opposite direction. (3) Even if they were enacted, I suspect that they would be only a temporary solution. I believe a duty to die would probably soon reemerge.

Why would it reemerge? We can begin to see why by noting that a widespread duty to die is a fairly recent phenomenon. It is largely the creation of the triumphs of medical progress. The successes of medicine enable us to live longer, even with serious illnesses.

Consider just one example. As recently as 60 years ago, those who were bedridden for a long time usually caught pneumonia. Since pneumonia often could not be successfully treated without respirators and effective antibiotics, bedridden people died. Because very sick or debilitated people died anyway—despite everything that medicine could offer—a duty to die was rare. Better medical treatments are a good thing. Who would want to be without them? But better medical treatments bring perplexing new moral problems and new responsibilities with them. This is what I have called the dark side of medical progress.

We should not expect medical progress to halt right now. The treatments for most diseases will almost certainly continue to improve. But these new and better treatments are almost always more expensive—usually both in financial terms and also in terms of care-giving. (1) As medicine progresses, most of us are likely to be able to benefit from more and more costly medical treatments. (2) As we improve treatment of diseases and lengthen our lifespans, we also increase the time during which we will live with chronic illness, debility, and/or dementia. As a result, medical progress also leaves more and more of us facing longer and longer periods of debility or dementia in which we will require more and more care from others.

Are these increasing burdens sustainable for a society? Justifiable? In the short run, yes. But in the longer run, I think not.

So even if we could summon the political and social will to do it, a decision to provide care collectively would very likely only buy us temporary relief from a duty to die. Medical progress will almost certainly overwhelm our social will—perhaps even our social ability—to pay for all needed medical treatments for everyone and also for care needed by all debilitated, demented, or chronically ill citizens. A finite world with finite resources seems to preclude indefinitely increasing socially provided payment for health care.

As health care costs continue to escalate, pressure to "save money" by externalizing the costs of health care would surely reemerge. We would then find our health care system beginning to do exactly what it is now doing—requiring families both to pay more and to bear more of the burdens of caring for the chronically ill and dying. We would eventually begin again to discharge people from hospitals "quicker and sicker," forcing families to provide the care they need. We would begin again to limit collective payment for institutional care for the debilitated, demented, and chronically ill. As these burdens of illness and debility on families increase, the likelihood that a person will face a duty to die increases, as well.

That is why I believe a duty to die would soon reemerge. It would probably reemerge even if we had all the collective good will in the world. Which we do not. I believe a duty to die is fairly common right now. Due both to lack of collective will and to medical progress, I believe a duty to die will be much more common 20 or 30 years from now—when it will be more grippingly relevant to most of us. We need to prepare ourselves, both individually and collectively, for this eventuality. We are not prepared. It will not be easy to get prepared. We had better start preparing now rather than hoping we will decide collectively to buy our way out of a duty to die.

DUTIES TO SELF AND DUTIES TO OTHERS

And on the much more intimate level of personal decisions, I must decide what I will do if our society does not reform itself in a way that eliminates the crushing burdens of serious illness on families or if it is unable to sustain this effort. In those very likely scenarios, what ought I to do? If the futures of my loved ones are not to be compromised by my illnesses, old age, and death, it will probably be up to me to see that this does not happen. Then a responsible death will sometimes involve a responsibility to decline medical treatments. I believe it may even involve a responsibility to take my own life.

In closing, then, let us return to the intimate, personal level on which my reflections center. When I advocate a duty to die, I begin with myself, with concern about my own loved ones. For me, the duty to die is, first of all, quite possibly my own duty, not someone else's. It is my own responsibilities that I most need to think about. But I invite you to think about yourself and your loved ones, too. For I believe a duty to die must, in the end, always be personal—self-recognized, self-imposed, and self-enforced.

Those who do not accept a duty to die evidently believe it is not irresponsible for me to force my wife or children to care for me in a debilitated or demented state for 6 or 8 years. That happens all the time. If better treatments were available that would slow the progress of my diseases, would it likewise be permissible to force my wife and children to care for me for 15 or 20 years?

After having lived a very good life myself, is there no moral reason why I must not—if I just want to live longer—preclude them from having a life anywhere near as good as mine? Of all the things that may be worth laying down my life for, the well-being of my loved ones is surely one. Sometimes, so far as I can see, this is the only loving thing to do.

Churchill asks us to consider what is involved in a responsible death and takes steps toward important parts of the answer. He reminds us of the long tradition of great and good people who have laid down their lives when conditions forced them to choose between their personal integrity and life itself.

The duty to self that Churchill discusses, the duty to family that I consider, and an expression of love are often, perhaps even usually, linked. If I see myself as the kind of person who is intimately connected with the ones I love and who love me, I will not want to extend my own life if I can do so only by leaving my loved ones with much poorer lives of their own. A duty to die then becomes not only an injunction to faithfulness to my loved ones, but also an act of faithfulness to myself and an expression of the loves that have been the center of my life. I will want to reaffirm my connection with my loved ones in my dying, as I have in my living. That will also be to affirm my sense of who I am and endow the end of my life with meaning. By contrast, my dying will be impoverished if I live and then die with the awareness that I have impoverished my loved ones and their lives in order to extend my own life a little longer.

It does not surprise me, then, that so many Americans of all ages report that they do not want to live if they become a burden to their loved ones. Yet many people end up becoming precisely the burden they feared they would. This may be because they believe they have no choice. In any case, their desire not to be a burden is routinely ignored by doctors and especially in health care facilities. As a result, those in institutions may well have no choice. People are also often told that ethically they have no choice, for it is wrong to take steps to end your life.

I believe I have choices. A whole range of possible deaths opens out before me and my choices will probably help shape the death that is mine. As one who has choices, I bear the responsibility, but also the opportunity to affirm my sense of myself and my loyalty to my loved ones. Like many others, it is critical to my identity and integrity that I am not selfish or self-centered and that I weigh carefully the needs of my loved ones (at least them!) in my dying as well as in my living. I want to contribute to their lives, certainly not impoverish them. I hope for them even better lives than I have lived and I want to help make that hope a reality. I hope I can reaffirm these values in my approach to the end of my life. I hope that I will be able to die in a way that does not compromise *both* my self and the lives of my loved ones.

Each of us will age, become ill, and die, duty to die or no. We know that we will die. If we have families and if we are loved, our approaching illness, debility, dementia, and death will affect more than just ourselves—in very important ways. We know that, too. For those who know such things, surely a good death must be a responsible death. Let us think together about how we can meet advancing age, illness, and death responsibly.

Notes

1. The *Encyclopedia of Philosophy* entry on "duty" does not even mention the word "rights," and the entry on "rights" explicitly states, "there are some duties, such as the duty of beneficence, where no one has a corresponding right to demand that they be performed" (Paul Edwards, editor-in-chief. *Encyclopedia of Philosophy*. New York: Macmillan, 1996. Vol. 7, 196). The entry on "rights" also points out that discussions of duty proceeded for centuries before the concept of rights became popular. Finally, Kant, a philosopher of duty if ever there was one, distinguishes negative from positive duties and points out that generally, no rights correspond to the latter. (For a discussion of Kant's use of this distinction, see Roger J. Sullivan, *Kant's Moral Theory*. Cambridge: Cambridge University Press, 1989.)

2. Traditional medicine and traditional medical ethics had the effect of removing responsibility from patients by removing the freedom. Traditionally, physicians made the decisions for their patients. If the doctor makes all the important decisions, she—rather than the patient—bears the responsibility for those decisions. But the traditional codes of medical ethics (though perhaps not the traditional practice of medicine) construed the physicians responsibility too narrowly—to promote the well-being of the patient. To the extent that physicians bear the responsibility for treatment decisions, they must not see themselves as patient advocates.

3. Strictly speaking, even medical vitalism will not justify the view that there are no limits to what families should do to care for a seriously ill or dying family member. Long-term caregiving often ruins the health of the caregiver and thereby shortens her life. So even if longer life were the highest value, there would be limits. The desire of a terminally ill family member to live longer would still not justify destroying the health of the caregiver; for the reduction in the lifespan of the caregiver would often be too great for a medical vitalist to sanction.

4. The Institute for Continued Learning, a group of senior citizens, compiled a list of responsibilities of those facing the end of life. I think it is a remarkable list and have included it in the Afterword to this volume. I consider it an excellent place to begin discussion of the various dimensions of a responsible approach to death.

5. These are some, but not all, of the relevant familial factors that I believe shape the responsibilities of the seriously ill: Their responsibilities depend on the resources—emotional

strength and resiliency, physical health, emotional support network, and financial situation—of the other members of the family. They depend on how many family members are able and willing to share the burdens of caregiving. They depend on the values, hopes, and dreams of other family members. They depend on many details of the family history—not only on the values to which they have been committed, but also on how various members have treated each other, who has made sacrifices for whom, what misfortunes have befallen various members of the family, and how family decisions have been made in the past.

6. Joanne Lynn, and James Childress. "Must Patients Always be Given Food and Water?" *Hastings Center Report* 13 (October 1983): 17–21. Joanne Lynn, ed. *By No Extraordinary Means.* Bloomington: Indiana UP, 1986.

7. Daniel Callahan. *The Troubled Dream of Life.* Washington, DC: Georgetown UP, 1994.

8. If the SUPPORT study of the economic impact of serious illness on families is anywhere close to correct, tens of thousands of families are impoverished each year. Kenneth E. Covinsky, et al. "The Impact of Serious Illness on Patients' Families." *Journal of the American Medical Association* 272 (1994): 1839–44.

9. Of course, this renewed emphasis on individual responsibility simultaneously makes it more likely that those of us who are relatively wealthy will be able to purchase personal exemption from a duty to die. Those who can afford to purchase extended care insurance can buy exemption for themselves. Those who can afford really first-rate health insurance also decrease their odds of personally facing a duty to die. Thus, CEOs and members of congress need face no duty to die. But most of us cannot individually afford to purchase exemption in these ways. ("Poor man's blood" in yet another guise!)

10. I have said very clearly that decisions about who has a duty to die will have to be very particular and contextual. Health care plans simply do not have the information required to decide that someone has a duty to die. Besides, on a more practical level, cutting payment for medical services and long-term care would probably increase the number of people who face a duty to die rather than reduce it. I wonder whether an insurance plan or government agency could afford to be recognized as doing that.

Afterword

Family Responses

What would a duty to die do to families? This is a critically important question to which we do not have the answer. The idea is still far too new and also too confined within its academic birthplace. Undoubtedly, it would have different effects in different families—even happy families are not all alike. I decided to ask *my* family. Unlike most people, they have been living for several years now with the knowledge that one of their loved ones honestly believes that he might one day have a duty to die . . . for them.

I asked my wife, Mary, and my sons, Bill and Jay, if they would write their personal responses to my essay, "Is There a Duty to Die?" Their responses follow. Mary and I have discussed the idea at length, at least in the abstract—she helped me write this and the other essays in this volume. I have never discussed either the essay or the idea with Bill or Jay. I did not talk with any of my family about their responses while they were writing.

Granted, the idea that I might have a duty to die is probably still somewhat remote for them. As far as any of us knows, I have no serious illnesses . . . yet. But the idea has been broached, and, once broached, it cannot be without ramifications.

The memory is an old one now, and if I were the more dramatic sort I might call it chilling. It is this: I am in the living room with my mother and father, reading a book of those dreadfully somber questions designed to provoke *real* conversation whenever such conversation is in short supply—a spot of soul-searching when the ballscores fail to satisfy.

I remember being struck by a particular question and, turning to face my parents, asking it aloud. "Would you like to know the precise date and time of your death?" To me the question spoke of all sorts of fanciful possibilities: how would we live our lives differently if we knew exactly when we would die? What a strange notion.

My father's response was more practical. "I plan to." he said. He formed a pistol with his fingers and drew it to his head. Smiling, he pulled the trigger. End of memory.

It goes without saying that I banished the thought to the back caverns of my brain at the first opportunity, but as his son I can tell you that the duty to die is not an idea my father cooked up at his desk some dark December morning when trying to think of how to get published in the finest journals. No, it's been with him for some time, an idea he's clearly stoked over the years, refined and revised, and only now been able to get down on paper. But those who know him well heard it long ago.

Now, my father is not in general a grim man, and to this day he enjoys a Ralph Stanley record and a plate of barbecue as well as any man, but for years he has been less than elusive about premeditated suicide. (Here I'll gladly confirm my father's contention that he is not "idiosyncratic, morbid, mentally ill, or morally perverse." Sometimes he doesn't match his clothes too well, but give the guy a break.) Some years later the pistol was replaced—too messy, I suppose—by the romance of hypothermia. He would simply walk into the woods on a very cold day, lie down, and wait. He had heard it was a peaceful, almost euphoric death. (What the heck, I thought, why not go over Niagara Falls in a wooden barrel, if you want to do it right?)

His dabblings were not limited to chilling gestures and offhand remarks: Whenever he brought up the idea of premeditated suicide, he was careful to talk about the choices and circumstances that might lead to such a final act. An honest effort, I'll admit, but each time he advanced the subject I was quick to dismiss it with a cough and nervous laugh and to ask him whether he thought the Colts had the running game to make the playoffs this year, and, since we're on the subject, how 'bout them Tennessee Volunteers? Go Big Orange.

But now my old man has really done it. He's gone and published the whole mess, first in a journal, now in a book, and it's become increasingly clear I won't be able to ignore the question forever. Looks like I'll be dragged smack into the heart of the debate, and by God one of these days—we haven't done it yet—we'll have to sit down, as a family, show our cards, and talk about *why* and *when* and *if*. The conversation is sure to be excruciating. Could have been avoided at one time, but can't now. I couldn't be more grateful.

My first emotion upon reading my father's article was *fear*. Fear that my father would feel the duty to die *too early*: Aged, aching, a little tired perhaps, holding a degenerative diagnosis in his hand, he would call up one day and tell me he had decided it was his time to go. And I fear that, however strong my protest, he would not be swayed. He would end his life, not only before *he* wanted to, but before *I* wanted him to.

Is this fear of a bad decision, or just a fear of my father's death? If it is the latter, there's no recourse. One of these days, by his own hand or not, my father is going to die, and that day will be one of terrible sadness. I fear that loss, I hate to hear my father talk about it, and I cannot read "Is There a Duty to Die?" without that fear in my throat. But that loss, as he points out, cannot be avoided, only postponed. It will come, and my father is clearly concerned that it come at the right time. I am proud of him for his strength to ask difficult questions, and I know he will not go blindly into that dark night.

But fear of a bad decision worries me also. "Given our society's reluctance to permit physicians, let alone family members, to perform aid-in-dying," my father writes, "I believe I may well have a duty to end my life when I can see mental incapacity on the horizon." I know by this that my father doesn't mean that the first time he forgets the milk at the grocery store he's coming home to off himself—if that had been the case, he'd barely have seen me out of diapers. But I do worry that he will come to consider himself a burden long before I do. (Indeed, I believe many older folks consider themselves burdens when their family does not.) I worry that we will not agree upon when he has a duty to die, or indeed if he will ever have such a duty. Ours will be a difference of *perspective*: he will not want to burden me; I will not want to lose my father, however great the burden. I want him to know that he could never be a burden to me, and at this distance, I can't fathom he would.

But he could. In my honest moments I admit as much. My father writes that we can now "survive longer than we can take care of ourselves, longer than we know what to do with ourselves, *longer than we even* are *ourselves*" (emphasis mine). And I agree that it happens that people sometimes outlive themselves. I can imagine my father bedridden, delusional, terminally ill, not himself, suspended in a thoughtless haze, and I know that no one in the family would want that end. And as dizzying as the thought is, there's a strange comfort in the knowledge that we might never have to see that end, that my father might choose to die before things reach that stage.

But would it ever be his *duty* to die? In his article, my father writes that the duty to die is based largely upon the sacrifices that your loved ones will have to make if you keep on living. He is talking, then, about me. Would I ever agree, morally, that my father has a *duty* to die so that my life will be more full? That my rights supersede his own in this, the most important of decisions? It seems unspeakably selfish to even entertain the notion. (Would my father ever agree that it was his father's duty to die? Would my sons ever agree that it was mine?)

Only when I flip the equation can I make much sense of it. While it's hard to imagine my father being a burden, it's easier to imagine myself being a burden to *my* children, when my own time comes. It is easier for me to imagine *myself* having a duty to die than it is to imagine my father having a duty to die. It is not that I am noble, or selfless, or rich with virtue. I suspect anyone would answer the same way. It is simply too difficult to condemn someone to death, whatever sacrifices lie in wait. I could never decide it was my father's duty to die; only he could make that decision. We could talk about it and fight and spit and scratch and scream and hug and laugh and cry, and in the end the difference would be this: he would know how I felt when it came time for him to make his decision.

And if we disagree? It is easy to imagine such a scenario, and that is what I fear. Adding up the options, my father may believe he has a duty to die, even if he would prefer to live. Adding up the same options, his family may believe he does not. Who decides? Would an honest discussion provoke agreement, or would it simply be the last great fight of our lives together? If my father, citing duty, ends his life before I feel his time has come, how will I respond? I hope I do not have to answer that question, but if I do, I hope we will have talked enough that I can answer it peaceably. I hope that I will understand his decision, and his reasons for making it, even if I disagree with it. I hope that everyone in our family can say the same. In the meantime, if he heads for the woods on a cold day, I'll make sure he has an extra sweater.

—Jay Hardwig

I am writing this response to my father's article "Is There a Duty to Die?" because throughout the essay he stresses the importance of family dialogue when talking about a duty to die. As he says in the article, "I believe in family decisions." So, in a very real sense, his writings cannot be seen as solely his ideas, his works: they affect us—his family and loved ones. This, then, is my reaction to his ideas, expressing how I see them influencing us as a family that might one day have to discuss the very issues he sets forth in this article.

Every family has its legends, the unforgettable stories in which myth and fact are woven together into the fabric of history. I remember one such legend especially clearly: It has stuck in my mind since the day I first heard my father tell it. The story begins with a tragedy—my great-grandfather (my father's grandfather) suffered a severe heart attack. Although he survived the attack, he was extremely weak and his doctor ordered him to remain in bed for weeks if not months. (The accuracy of the details no longer matters much, as the facts of my great-grandfather's life have been converted into the narratives with which my family makes sense of our existence, our past.) As my dad tells the story, my great-grandfather was deeply concerned with becoming a burden to the family. He believed that the family could not survive without his income, and he feared that their potential for earning a living would be tied up in caring for him. It is here that the story becomes legend: In order to ease the financial burden, my great-grandfather pulled his wrecked body out of bed, hobbled to the staircase and with a look of triumphant defiance on his face (so the story goes) hurled himself down the staircase, thus alleviating the family of the responsibility to care for him and allowing them to collect his life insurance and move on with their lives.

This is the part of the story that has fascinated me since my childhood. My great-grandfather's suicide may have been an act of unselfish thoughtfulness, heroism even (he apparently thought so), but mixed in with this heroism is for me a profound horror. Did this man think that money was the most important and only contribution he could provide his family? Could he not conceive of any way he could be an integral and vital part of the family if he no longer had the ability to support them financially? Was killing himself the most meaningful act he could envision doing for his family?

I remember equally clearly my father's reaction to the story. He seemed to identify with my grandfather (the deceased man's young son) and always ended the story with a comment about how strange it was to make this decision solely a financial one. In my dad's eyes (as least as he saw things several years ago), this act was wrong—heroic perhaps, but a misplaced heroism that oddly defined one's worth in dollars and cents.

I bring up this story because when my father first told me his ideas about a *duty to die,* I recalled this story and wondered how he could believe in a duty to die when he was so clearly opposed to what my great-grandfather saw as a dutiful death. It seemed to me as though his personal reaction to a family crisis was inconsistent with his theoretical ideas about abstract illnesses. But as I read and reread his article, I began to believe that his reaction to his grandfather's story and his belief in a duty to die were consistent with one another. After all, much of "Is There a Duty to Die?" deals with the importance of an in-depth communication with loved ones about this duty. Each family, he writes, "must be allowed to speak for themselves about the burdens [an ill person's] life imposes on them and how they feel about bearing those burdens." There is certainly no mention of a family discussion in the legend of my great-grandfather. Also, the article emphasizes that there are often ways of contributing to a family that offset the financial burdens the ill person may create. "If my loved ones are truly benefitting from coping with my illness or debility, I have no duty to die based on burdens to them." In short, my great-grandfather seemed to be acting in accordance with what my father has called "the individualistic fantasy." Even though he perceived a duty to die instead of a desperate need to prolong life, my great-grandfather came to this decision by himself, without consulting the family and without discussing what burden he would be placing on them.

With this said, I would like to return to my belief that during the telling of my great-grandfather's story my father identified with his father (the child experiencing the loss of a loved one), because for me the *duty to die* takes on a very different reality for the caregiver than it does for the dying or debilitated subject. I wonder if my father might have different reactions to his grandfather's death and his own duty to die in part because he identifies with the survivor in one situation (his grandfather's death) and the dying person in the other (his own duty to die). In any case, we need to recognize that while the caregivers and the debilitated/ill person may be speaking of the same subject, they are approaching it from vastly different directions. If this contract between a dying person and his/her loved ones is to be honest and effective, there must be a clear understanding about when this duty to die becomes relevant and indeed necessary. In the article, my father discusses his realization that family conversations about the topic will not always produce truthful discussions: There are times when caregivers will feel an overwhelming burden but will not admit it: "[M]any families seem unable to talk about death at all, much less a duty to die." In this case, "Is There a Duty to Die?" suggests that you look for "behavioral clues"—financial and physical conditions, anxiety—to help make your decision.

As the child of someone who espouses the belief in a duty to die, this idea bothers me. What frightens me the most about my father's responsibility to die lies in his acknowledgment that he may have to interpret empirically these "clues" in order to make a responsible decision. Do I want my father to base the biggest decision of his life on appearances? Are my "behavioral clues" an adequate means of determining the extent to which my ill father would be a burden?

Obviously, these questions hinge upon how we determine and define what a burden is. I can easily imagine a scenario in which my father would feel as if he is being an excessive burden, while his loved ones would not. As he recognizes in the article, there are some burdens that are not necessarily negative, even if they cause financial and emotional strain. The loved ones of a dying person often feel the need/responsibility/duty to give to (and sacrifice for) a dying person in part because of how much that person gave while he/she was healthy. I'm not talking about a self-effacing sacrifice or a foolish loyalty, but a real need to help others as you have been helped. I wonder whether a dying person can accurately surmise these needs and whether the caregivers are capable of adequately expressing them. What we are dealing with then is the difference between the *needs* of the caregivers and these *needs as perceived* by the dying person. By no means do I see these two ideas as necessarily correlating. If my father were dying and felt like a burden although his loved ones did not feel he was, what would we do? What would he do?

As the article mentions, truthful conversations between family members help define what a burden means to each family. These discussions might be painful and difficult, but they are an essential part of the commitment to a duty to die. However, honesty would seem to be a scarce commodity when a family is faced with an impending death. Could a caregiver honestly tell a dying loved one that he/she has become a burden? Conversely, could the dying person adequately judge whether a loved one is honest in his or her expression of what a "burden" constitutes?" Perhaps *honesty* is not the central issue within these conversations (in fact, I'm not sure how I'd define honesty in these circumstances): rather, it seems to me that it is a matter of *perspective*. Can a person gain the necessary perspective to make these decisions and voice them clearly when a loved one is dying? Can the dying person gain the necessary perspective to interpret the "behavior clues" of a loved one who is watching him/her die? As I said before, I can easily imagine my father feeling as though he were a burden to his caregivers in degrees much greater than our family would actually feel this burden or even perceive it as a burden. I'm not sure these are issues that we could honestly deal with around a hospital bed: there are too many variables, too many emotions.

I believe that in order even to begin to get the perspective necessary to approach these questions and define what we mean by a "burden," our family must discuss these issues before a debilitating illness or accident occurs. As "Is There a Duty to Die?" mentions, without question, a large part of this dialogue would involve an interrogation of what death and dying mean to each of us. These discussions would be heart-wrenching, as the definitions of an unacceptable burden and a meaningful death would have to be hammered out in unpleasant detail. While I believe discussing these ideas before the onset of a family crisis would help make these decisions slightly less traumatic for our family and would perhaps make "behavioral clues" a little less determining (or more easily interpretable), it will never be easy. I wonder if it is *ever* possible, even when discussing an abstract debilitation in the undetermined future, for most families to get the necessary perspective to address these questions in a forthright manner. How do we decide what is a reasonable sacrifice? Does reason even help in the discussion about our commitment to loved ones?

As I write this, I wonder if my dad had us in mind when he wrote that "many families seem unable to talk about death . . . much less a duty to die." It occurs to me that we have never had much discussion about death, at least the death of people we love. I know that he feels he may someday have a duty to die and that he does not want his life unnaturally prolonged by machines, but we've never really discussed the nuts and bolts of how we/he would decide what constitutes an unacceptable burden. Perhaps the most telling indication of how difficult these conversations will be is that even though we've discussed "the duty to die" several times in recent months, and even though my great-grandfather's suicide/death has entered into these conversations, I still don't know how my father feels about this suicide now. Has he changed his opinion about his grandfather's actions as his thoughts on a duty to die have evolved? I don't know the answer to this question. Perhaps the fact that I'm not sure how Dad would see his grandfather's death today demonstrates a lack of communication about death and dying *in our family*. If so, I suspect we are not alone. This silence, however, does not in my mind undermine the validity of the points made in "Is There a Duty to Die?" (In fact, I end this response agreeing with the principal thrust of the argument.) Rather, this silence emphasizes to me that we, as a family, have some very distressing conversations in our not-too-distant future—conversations that may not be enjoyable (or even completely honest), but are truly vital.

—Bill Hardwig

I should begin with some background. John and I are both in our 50s: He's four years older than I. We've known each other a long time— more than 20 years—and over that time we've become increasingly involved with each other. However, as I write this in late winter of 1999, we've been married less than two years. Both of us were married before, but whereas my first marriage ended many years ago and resulted in no children, John's lasted much longer and resulted in Bill and Jay.

This leads to my first point, one that John has alluded to in several of his articles. What counts as a "family" is neither clear nor static. John and I have been constituting our own "family of two" over some time: now, for me, that family is expanding to include his sons and their wives. John and I also have our "birth" families—parents, siblings and their spouses, nieces and nephews, etc.—and those birth families are evolving as well. Mine, in fact, is going through an upheaval. More on that later.

Back to the first point: Who should a patient take into consideration when she wrestles with the thought that she may have a duty to die? And—a harder question yet—whose views should she actively seek, individually or through a family conversation, about that possible duty? These are all procedural questions: They're not intended to refute John's main point. Perhaps the answers to these proce-dural questions will be obvious when a patient is faced with a possi-ble duty to die. But perhaps not.

Someone may be left out of the family conversation, inadver-tently or knowingly—for example, if he's not around or has never been easy to talk with. The likely result would be that the patient (and other family members) wouldn't adequately understand his views, and vice versa. Or if the patient consulted him as an after-thought only, the likely result would be to inflict a lasting hurt, a sense of his inconsequence in the patient's life and the life of the fam-ily. Again, I'm not trying to contradict John here: I'm simply empha-sizing that these family conversations will be delicate matters—mat-ters that might be difficult to think through and orchestrate even under normal circumstances but will be especially difficult if you are contemplating a duty to die.

Related to the question of who constitutes the family is a second point: All members of the family are not equal regarding a patient's possible duty to die; some members' interests and concerns will (or should) weigh more heavily than others. If a patient's spouse is alive and reasonably well, it is likely that the spouse will have the greatest burden of care for the patient—physically, emotionally, and finan-cially. The issue of who will have the greatest burden of care is cen-tral to the "weighting" question. But should the views of that family member (typically, the spouse) on the patient's duty to die then trump the views of all other family members? Not necessarily. The spouse could affirm the patient's duty to die and refuse to be a care-giver: the other family members might then decide to pick up the slack (although, under present law, the financial burden would still fall mainly on the spouse). Or, in a more plausible scenario, the spouse could repudiate the patient's duty to die and shoulder the caregiving responsibilities but then become ill or die himself, in which case the other family members would be left with some responsibilities for the patient. The extent to which other, non-spousal family members have responsibilities for the patient involves matters of the heart as well as practical matters, and the two can eas-ily become intertwined.

How is the patient to sort all this out? With difficulty, undoubt-edly. My own strongly held opinion is that the lighter the burden of the patient's continued life on a family member, the less weight that family member should have in dissuading a patient from a duty to die. Yet I can easily imagine situations in which grown children would be appalled at the idea of their parent killing herself, even though it made painful good sense to those on the daily scene. This suggests that, if the patient has some time in which to reach and then execute a decision to die, part of that time should be spent trying to bring peace to those family members least able to accept the patient's death. To do so would not be easy and might involve acts of courage: opening up discussion, not only of the patient's coming death, but also of unresolved old wounds. These would be acts of emotional generosity at a time when, understandably, a patient might feel most inclined to mentally withdraw from the world.

I want to switch now to a different and more personal point. You've heard in what John has written—as well as in his sons' essays—about the experiences in his paternal lineage: the death of his father at 60 because of a heart attack; the death (or suicide) of his grandfather, also at a relatively young age and also because of a heart attack. This family history has, I think, colored the way in which John thinks about a duty to die. He reflects upon *his* possible duty to die, not upon mine or Bill's or Jay's. He assumes he'll go (or need to go) first. I agree with most of what he has said about a duty to die, but I'd argue that his thinking may be somewhat clouded by this possibly counterfactual perspective. He focuses on the patient; he needs to explore further the perspective of a patient's family member.

For who can say who will first have a possible duty to die? To illustrate this point, I'll return to what's happening with my birth family. My father, now 82, is five years older than my mother. They've been married for 56 years. I'm fairly certain that for most of those years, dad assumed that he would die before mom (another history of early paternal heart attacks). And both, I think, assumed that when they went, they would go quickly. There were heart attacks and little else on my mother's side of the family as well . . . or at least not until now. Now, my mother has terminal liver cancer (diagnosed one year ago) and my father has mid-stage Alzheimer's disease (first apparent about six years ago). They're still living in their own home in Vermont, 300 miles from the nearest of their four children. Dad never discussed his condition at length with anyone, including his wife (and is now unable to); Mom has been forthright about her disease and its prognosis. They've provided well for themselves, so money is not an issue. Nor does either parent necessarily have a duty to die.

I relate this story to illustrate three messages. First, conversations about a duty to die should begin early and in the abstract, well before anyone is faced with an actual possible duty to die. Family members need to become accustomed to the topic before it becomes palpably real. They also need to explore their feelings with (and have their positions challenged by) other family members. All family members need not be present, sitting around the dinner table at Thanksgiving, for these abstract conversations to begin. In our family (John's and mine), he has launched the topic. It's now up to all of us to give it silent and spoken thought.

Second, in these early, abstract discussions about a possible duty to die, we should not make assumptions about who will have the duty or about what our stations in life will be in other respects. Instead, we should explore different situations without committing ourselves to positions that we will be held to if an actual occasion arises.

And third, while money can help a great deal, it does not necessarily buy us out of making decisions about death. Granted, money can greatly lighten the burden a patient might otherwise impose, but choosing death may still be the best decision—not out of a grim sense of duty, but because it may be the wise and honorable thing to do, for ourselves as well as for those closest to us.

—Mary English

A Responsible Death—Getting the Discussion Started

I have always been interested in talking with seniors about the end of life. But I've been a little reluctant, too—it's taboo to talk with seniors about dying, partly because it might seem to suggest that the elderly have nothing left to do but die. Still, the elderly know that they may not have all that long to live. Surely, many of them think about the end of life. Taboo or not, it cannot really make sense to refrain from asking seniors what they think about the end of life.

So, when invited to talk to The Institute for Continued Learning, a seniors' organization dedicated to providing educational opportunities for its members, I seized the opportunity. I told the group that I wanted to talk with them about a responsible death. I talked very briefly about autonomy and responsibility. (They all quickly agreed that autonomy involves responsibility.) I said that there are important responsibilities of *others*, particularly family members, to the aged, the infirm, the ill, and the dying. But today, I wanted them to tell me what they think are the responsibilities of those facing the end of life.

I think they came up with a remarkable list. We had only 45 minutes for our discussion, so we could not spend a lot of time talking about each proposed responsibility. But all were at least briefly discussed. Not everyone present agreed with every item on the list they formulated. But there was considerable consensus about many of them, as well as comments like, "I'd better start doing that."

At the end of our brief discussion, one women came up to me and said, "My husband passed away 3 weeks ago. I just want you to know how comforting and helpful this discussion has been to me."

The list of responsibilities these seniors formulated is not uncontroversial. But it was evident that each represents the deeply held conviction of someone who is thoughtfully facing the end of life. Each is worthy of serious consideration. The list of responsibilities they formulated strikes me as an excellent starting point for moral discussion of our responsibilities at the end of life. I offer it as such.

Responsibilities of Those Facing the End of Life

The following was formulated by the Institute for Continued Learning, Johnson City, Tennessee, November 5, 1998. The Institute for Continued Learning is a group of seniors who meet regularly to participate in educational events and programs. They are all retired. The youngest member of the group is 55 years old. Most are in their 70s.

1. Talk with your family about death.

2. Die in a way that will leave your family in the best position. (A discussion followed about whether there is a responsibility to commit suicide. Some think there is.)

3. Make a will.

4. Discuss death and dying while you are well. Renew this discussion periodically.

5. Don't live so long that your loved ones will wish you were dead. (Discussion followed of the comment one member had heard from a friend: "I wish my mother had died while I still loved her.")

6. Don't insist on personal care. Don't ever say, "Never put me in a nursing home." If you've said that, retract it and apologize.

7. Review the life you have shared, set things right, and ask for forgiveness from your loved ones.

8. Make a living will.

9. Don't leave to others decisions that will cause guilt.

10. Teach your spouse and inform your children about your finances.

11. Do things to minimize disagreements and conflicts among your survivors.

12. If you decide on suicide, be considerate of those who will find your body.

13. Put all your assets in both names . . . or separate them. Review this.

14. Write an obituary, make funeral and burial plans. Address the issue of donation of your body.

15. Talk with your loved ones about what they will do after you're dead and about how their lives will be without you. This will give them permission to go on to full lives after you're dead.

16. Teach household responsibilities to ensure that your spouse has competencies he or she will need when you are dead. (In discussion, many felt the husband should cook, clean, and do the wash for a couple of months while the wife pays the bills, gets the car serviced, and takes care of the house/yard.)

17. Help your spouse achieve enough independence and enough of a life of his or her own to live happily without you.

18. Tell your story (partly as a way of accomplishing all of this).

Contributors

DANIEL CALLAHAN is the director of international programs at the Hastings Center, and the author, most recently, of *False Hopes*, Simon and Schuster, 1998.

LARRY R. CHURCHILL is professor of social medicine at the University of North Carolina at Chapel Hill, where he teaches ethics and humanities. His most recent books are *Self-Interest and Universal Health Care*, Harvard. Press, 1994, and *The Social Medicine Reader* (co-editor), Duke. Press, 1997.

FELICIA COHN is a senior scientist with the Center to Improve Care of the Dying and the director of the Program in Bioethics at the George Washington University Medical Center. She teaches and does research on end-of-life care, the clinician-patient relationship, and clinical ethics consultation.

NAT HENTOFF is a journalist who writes a weekly column for *Village Voice* and columns for *The Washington Post* that are syndicated in over 200 newspapers. He has written extensively on the Bill of Rights, especially the freedom of speech.

JOANNE LYNN is director of the Center to Improve Care of the Dying, and professor of health care sciences at the George Washington University Medical Center. Dr. Lynn is also president of Americans for Better Care of the Dying.

Index

A

Abimelech, suicide of, 158, 163(n6)
abuse, definition of, 68–71
advocates, for patient, 5, 37–39, 65, 135(n3)
affirmation, role in personal relationships, 19
AIDS
  cures for, 120
  death as relief from, 83
  effects on patient's family, 31
  late death from, 97
ALS
  cure for, 120
  death as relief from, 83
altruism
  egoism compared to, 23
  motives of, 21
Alzheimer's disease, 197
  case history of patient with, 45, 47–49, 50, 51–52, 57
  duty to die and, 90, 129, 148, 158
  effects on patient's family, 31, 174
  effects on spouse, 67, 69–70, 74, 77, 87
Aquinas, Thomas, as opponent of suicide, 159, 160
Aristotle
  ethics of virtue of, 19
  "friendships of utility" of, 10–11
aspiration, ethics of, 25
Augustine of Hippo, as opponent of suicide, 159, 160
autobiographies
  alternatives to, 114–16
  clinical encounters and, 109–10
  epistemology of, 102–7
  ignorance in, 104
  innocent mistakes in, 104, 105
  lies in, 104, 106–7
  moral evaluation of, 110–14
  multiple, 107–8
  in narrative ethics, 101–17
  oppression imposed by, 113–14
  reliability of, 115–16
  self–deception in, 104, 105, 107, 108
autonomy
  of family, 41
  interpretation of, 37–38
  of patient, 29, 37–39, 42, 53, 64–65, 97–98, 116
  reinterpretation of, 116
  responsibility and, 166–68
  of terminally ill patient, 64

B

benevolence
  motives of, 21
  unacceptability in personal relationships, 22
"benevolence" model, of medical ethics, 35
best-interest standard, for proxy decisions, 46
bioethics
  emphasis on doctor-patient dyad, 4
  family-centered, 2, 166–67
  "patient-centered", 2–3, 4–5
  responsibility in, 166